About me!

Greetings! I'm KS Kamboh, a seasoned doctor with a penchant for helping people navigate the complex landscape of their health. With my stethoscope as a trusted sidekick, I've embarked on a medical journey that's taken me from the bustling clinics of Pakistan to the rolling green hills of Ireland and now to the heart of the NHS in the UK.

But beyond the titles and the degrees, what truly drives me is the desire to make a difference in the lives of individuals like you. You see, I've had the privilege of working with countless patients, each with their unique set of health challenges. It's these interactions that have shaped my perspective and motivated me to share my knowledge with the world.

My goal has always been to demystify the world of medicine, to bridge the gap between healthcare professionals and the individuals seeking answers and support. So, join me on this journey. Let's explore the intriguing realm of health together, where I promise to be your trusted companion, helping you make informed decisions about your well-being and offering a friendly hand in the often bewildering maze of healthcare. So, welcome to my world. It's a pleasure to meet you!

About this Book!

In crafting this narrative on asthma, I step into multiple roles – that of an experienced medical professional, a compassionate caregiver, and an individual intimately familiar with the challenges of managing asthma. What distinguishes this work is its departure from a mere compilation of clinical facts; it is, instead, a labor of devotion, a repository of insights gleaned from my encounters both within the medical realm and within the confines of my own family. Asthma, a multifaceted respiratory condition, serves as the focal point of our exploration. My objective is to demystify its complexities in a manner that resonates with clarity. I've walked in the shoes of a healthcare provider, articulating diagnosis to patients, and as a supportive family member navigating the undulating journey alongside those grappling with asthma. This distinct perspective positions me to address the substantive issues and queries that hold genuine significance.

From unraveling the root causes of asthma to elucidating the diagnostic journey, this work spans a comprehensive spectrum. It extends beyond mere understanding to delve deeply into the intricacies of asthma management, offering insights on treatment alternatives, post-management strategies, and the often-overlooked emotional support crucial to this expedition.

Within these pages, we'll navigate discussions on dietary considerations, exercise regimens, and lifestyle adjustments that can significantly impact the asthma journey. Throughout, you'll encounter a friendly, empathetic voice – mine – guiding you through each nuanced step.

Consider this work not just a book but a steadfast companion on your asthma expedition. Whether you are an individual contending with asthma, a dedicated caregiver, or someone intrigued by the intricacies of this respiratory condition, I stand ready to furnish the answers and support you seek. It transcends the confines of a mere literary creation; it's a guiding presence, a wellspring of solace, and a testament to the potency of knowledge and understanding. Welcome to this expedition – I'm eager to share it with you.

Table of Contents

Chapter 1

Understanding Asthma; General Information.

Imagine you're taking a stroll in the park on a sunny day, the air is crisp, and the birds are singing. Suddenly, you find it hard to catch your breath. Your chest tightens, and you begin to cough and wheeze. It feels like there's a weight on your chest, making it difficult to draw in air. If you've ever experienced this, you might be familiar with asthma.

1.What is Asthma?

Asthma is like having a picky guest in your lungs who decides to throw a party at the most inconvenient times. In simple terms, it's a chronic (meaning, it hangs around for a while) condition that affects your breathing. But don't worry, you're not alone – over 300 million people worldwide have asthma, and they're all navigating this respiratory rollercoaster.

The Marvelous Machine Called Lungs

To understand asthma, let's take a quick peek into the marvelous machine called lungs. Your lungs are like two spongy balloons residing in your chest, and they have a crucial job: helping you breathe. When you inhale, you're pulling in fresh air filled with life-enabling oxygen. The lungs then pass this oxygen into your bloodstream, providing fuel for your body's engine.

Now, imagine your lungs as a well-coordinated team of workers. Each worker has a specific task. One worker ensures the airways stay open and clear, while another makes sure that your lungs don't over inflate or collapse. It's a symphony of tasks happening effortlessly – until asthma decides to stir the waters.

A Dance of Inflammation and Tightening

In the world of asthma, there's a mischievous duo: inflammation and tightening. When you encounter a trigger (more on that later), your airways throw a bit of a tantrum. The walls of these air passages get irritated, swollen, and inflamed, making it harder for air to flow smoothly. It's like trying to sip a refreshing drink through a straw that someone squished – not the easiest task.

As if that's not enough, there's a second act to this asthma drama: tightening. The muscles around your airways decide to flex their muscles (literally), making the passages even narrower. It's like trying to squeeze through a narrow doorway while carrying a backpack – not the most comfortable experience.

The Trigger Game

Now, let's talk about triggers. Triggers are like the troublemakers at the asthma party. They can vary from person to person, but some common ones include pollen (the stuff that makes flowers pretty but can make your nose itch), pet dander (tiny particles from furry friends), dust mites (microscopic creatures living in your bedding), and even strong emotions or stress (yes, your lungs can be sensitive souls).

Think of triggers as the spark that lights the asthma fire. Identifying and avoiding these troublemakers is a crucial part of managing asthma. It's like playing hide-and-seek with things that make your lungs grumpy.

Asthma: Not One Size Fits All

One important thing to know about asthma is that it's not a one-size-fits-all condition. Just as people have different tastes in music or favorite ice cream flavors, asthma can manifest in various ways. Some may have occasional flare-ups, while others might deal with it more frequently. The key is to understand your unique asthma story and work with your healthcare team to manage it effectively.

Conclusion

In a nutshell, asthma is like having a rebellious orchestra in your lungs, playing a tune of inflammation and tightening when triggered by certain factors. Understanding your asthma and its triggers is the first step toward managing this condition and living a full, active life.

In the following chapters, we'll delve deeper into the world of asthma, exploring how to identify triggers, manage symptoms, and create a personalized asthma action plan. So, buckle up – your journey to mastering asthma has just begun!

2.How Does inflammation of airways affect your Asthma?

In the last chapter, we touched on the basics of asthma - the mischievous orchestra in your lungs and the triggers that set the stage for a respiratory rollercoaster. Now, let's take a closer look at a key player in this drama: inflammation.

The Sneaky Intruder: Inflammation Unveiled

Think of your airways as the highway for the breath of life. In a world without asthma, this highway is smooth and clear, allowing air to flow freely like a gentle breeze. But when asthma steps into the scene, it brings along a sneaky intruder: inflammation.

Picture inflammation as the uninvited guest at the asthma party. It's like a little mischief-maker causing a ruckus in the calm and orderly world of your airways. But what exactly is inflammation, and how does it throw a wrench into the breathing machinery?

The Inflammation Showdown

Inflammation is the body's way of responding to something it sees as a threat. It's like the alarm bell ringing in a medieval castle when enemies approach. In asthma, this response is triggered by things called irritants, which can range from pollen and dust to pet dander and even stress.

So, here's how the inflammation showdown unfolds: when these irritants make their entrance, your body's defense system kicks in. Cells release chemicals that make the walls of your airways throw a little fit – they swell up, get all red and irritated, and make it harder for air to pass through. It's like trying to drive a car through a road full of potholes – not the smoothest journey.

The Airway Red Carpet Turned Chaotic

In a non-asthma world, your airways are like a well-maintained red carpet, allowing air to glide in and out effortlessly. But when inflammation barges in, it's like the red carpet turns into a chaotic obstacle course. The once smooth path becomes bumpy and restricted, causing you to feel like you're breathing through a straw.

This inflammation-induced chaos is what leads to the classic symptoms of asthma – the wheezing, the coughing, and that feeling of tightness in your chest.

It's like your airways are throwing a protest, making it challenging for the air to take its leisurely stroll into your lungs.

Meet the Inflammation Squad: Cells and Chemicals

Now, let's meet the inflammation squad – the cells and chemicals that turn your airways into a drama-filled stage. Picture cells as the little workers in your body, each with a specific job. When inflammation kicks in, these workers release chemicals, like histamines and leukotrienes, into the mix.

Histamines are like the drama queens of inflammation. They cause the walls of your airways to swell and produce mucus, turning your once tidy air passages into a congested mess. It's like the cells are shouting, "Emergency! Let's batten down the hatches!" but forgetting to clean up after themselves.

Leukotrienes, on the other hand, are like the troublemakers who tighten the muscles around your airways. They add an extra layer of chaos by making it even more challenging for the air to find its way in. It's like they're playing a game of "How many obstacles can we throw in the airways today?"

The Domino Effect of Inflammation

Now, let's talk about the domino effect. Once inflammation starts its mischief, it can trigger a chain reaction. The irritated airways become more sensitive, and even small triggers that were once harmless can now set off a full-blown asthma episode.

It's like your lungs have become a little too touchy, reacting strongly to things that shouldn't cause much trouble. This domino effect is why understanding and managing inflammation are crucial steps in the asthma journey. It's like putting a fence around the mischievous guest at the asthma party – in this case, inflammation – to keep it from causing too much trouble.

Taming the Inflammation Beast

The good news is that we have tools to tame the inflammation beast. Medications known as anti-inflammatories can be superheroes in this story. They work to calm down the irritated airways, like a soothing lullaby for your respiratory system.

Inhaled corticosteroids, for example, are like the peacekeepers in the asthma world. They reduce the inflammation and help your airways return to their smoother, more open state. It's like sending the troublemaking inflammation squad on vacation, giving your lungs a break.

A Team Effort: You and Your Healthcare Squad

Understanding how inflammation affects your asthma is the first step in taking charge of your respiratory adventure. It's like having a map for the journey, showing you the twists and turns so you can navigate with confidence.

Remember, managing asthma is a team effort. You're not alone on this adventure. Your healthcare squad, including your doctor and other asthma experts, is here to guide you. Together, you can develop a plan to keep inflammation in check, ensuring that your airways stay clear for the smooth flow of that life-enabling breeze.

In the upcoming chapters, we'll dive deeper into the tools and strategies for managing inflammation, exploring lifestyle adjustments, and creating a personalized action plan for your unique asthma story. So, get ready for the next leg of the adventure – we're just getting started!

3.Who Gets Asthma?

We've covered the basics and danced with inflammation. Now, let's dive into a question many wonder about: Who gets asthma? Is it a selective club, or can anyone be handed the golden ticket to this wheezy party?

Asthma: No VIP Pass Required

Here's the good news – or maybe not-so-good news, depending on how you look at it: asthma doesn't play favorites. It's an equal-opportunity condition, and anyone can find themselves with an invite to the asthma shindig. Young or old, big or small, asthma has been known to knock on the doors of people from all walks of life.

The Mystery Behind the Invitations

While asthma doesn't discriminate, there are a few factors that might influence whether you get that golden ticket or not. Let's peel back the curtain and explore the mysteries behind the invitations:

1. **Family Ties:**

   - It turns out that genetics can play a role in your likelihood of joining the asthma club. If your parents or siblings have asthma, you might be more likely to get that golden ticket. But, and it's a big but, having asthma in the family doesn't guarantee you'll be part of the wheezy party.

2. **Environmental Exposures:**

   - Picture your surroundings as the setting for the asthma tale. If you live in an area with lots of air pollution, cigarette smoke, or industrial fumes, you might be at a higher risk of getting that golden ticket. It's like your environment is whispering to your lungs, and sometimes it's not saying the nicest things.

3. **Early Childhood Adventures:**

   - Your early years can shape your asthma destiny. Babies exposed to smoke, infections, or allergens in their first few years might have a higher chance of becoming asthma's plus-one. It's like the groundwork for the asthma adventure is laid in the early chapters of your life story.

4. **Allergies:**

- Imagine allergies as the prequel to asthma. If you're prone to allergies, your immune system might be a bit sensitive, increasing the likelihood of getting that coveted golden ticket. It's like the body's way of saying, "Hey, I'm sensitive to things, can asthma join the party too?"

5. **The Viral Intruders:**

- Viruses can be sneaky gatecrashers at the asthma party. Respiratory infections, especially in childhood, can sometimes pave the way for asthma to make its grand entrance. It's like the viruses are handing out flyers, inviting asthma to join the festivities.

6. **Exercise-Induced Asthma:**

- Now, here's an interesting twist. Some people get a special edition of the golden ticket called exercise-induced asthma. It's like your lungs decide to throw a little wheezy party whenever you decide to hit the gym or run around in the great outdoors.

Asthma's Sneaky Timing:

- Asthma can be a fashionably late guest or make its entrance early in life. Some people discover their asthma adventures as kids, while others might not experience it until adulthood. It's like asthma has its own schedule, surprising you when you least expect it.

No Crystal Ball:

- Here's the catch – we don't have a crystal ball to predict who gets the golden ticket. Sometimes, asthma shows up unannounced, and other times, it sits quietly in the background, waiting for the perfect moment to make an entrance.

Asthma Across the Globe:

Asthma is a world traveler; it's not bound by borders. People from different corners of the globe have experienced the wheezy notes of asthma. It can be found in bustling cities, serene suburbs, and even in the quiet countryside. The common thread is that asthma doesn't discriminate based on geography.

The Changing Guest List:
Asthma's guest list can change over time. Some people might outgrow their asthma adventures, especially if it started in childhood. Others might develop asthma later in life, seemingly out of the blue. It's like the guest list is constantly evolving, with new arrivals and departures.

Cultural Perspectives:
Asthma doesn't have a preferred cultural background. It's found in people of all races and ethnicities. However, how asthma is perceived and managed can vary across cultures. Understanding and respecting these cultural perspectives can be essential in providing effective asthma care.

Conclusion:
In the grand ballroom of health, asthma extends invitations without checking your background or credentials. It can affect anyone, whether you're a city dweller or live surrounded by fields and meadows. The key is to understand the factors that might increase the chances of getting that golden ticket and be prepared for the unexpected twists and turns in your asthma adventure.
Remember, having asthma doesn't define you. It's just one part of your unique story. In the upcoming chapters, we'll explore how to navigate the asthma adventure, regardless of when you received your golden ticket or what your asthma story looks like. So, get ready for more insights, tips, and strategies as we continue this wheezy journey together!

4.The Beginning - At What Age Does Asthma Start?

Asthma is like an unexpected visitor; it doesn't knock on the door before entering. But have you ever wondered at what age this uninvited guest tends to make its entrance? Let's embark on a journey to unravel the mysteries of when asthma often decides to show up in our lives.

The Early Years:

Picture this: a baby's first cry, the soft gurgles, and the adorable sneezes. It's a magical time, but even in these early days, asthma can sometimes make a subtle entrance. Yes, asthma can start as early as infancy. Don't worry, though; it's not common, and the symptoms are usually less dramatic than those in older children or adults.

Toddler Troubles:

As our little ones start to explore the world on wobbly legs, their curious minds and developing bodies may encounter asthma for the first time. Toddlers, typically between the ages of 2 and 5, can experience asthma symptoms. These might include bouts of coughing, especially at night, or wheezing during playtime. Remember, if you suspect asthma in your toddler, it's essential to consult with a healthcare professional for a proper diagnosis.

School-age Surprises:

As kids venture into the school-age years, asthma can decide to join the adventure. Between the ages of 6 and 12, children may start showing more noticeable signs of asthma. This could include shortness of breath, chest tightness, or coughing, particularly after physical activities or exposure to certain triggers.

Adolescence Awakens:

Ah, adolescence - a time of growth spurts, changing voices, and, for some, the debut of asthma symptoms. While asthma often begins in childhood, some individuals experience their first asthma symptoms during their teenage years. The hormonal changes and increased independence during adolescence can play a role in the onset of asthma or the exacerbation of existing symptoms.

Adult Onset:

Surprisingly, asthma can also make a grand entrance in adulthood. Yes, you heard it right - adults can develop asthma even if they've never experienced it before. This can happen due to a variety of factors, including exposure to new allergens, changes in the environment, or even certain infections.

The Golden Years:

Just when you thought you were in the clear, asthma might decide to stick around or make a comeback in the golden years. While it's less common for asthma to first appear in older adults, individuals who had asthma earlier in life may continue to experience symptoms as they age.

Why Does Asthma Choose Its Moment?

Now, you might be wondering, "Why does asthma decide to make an entrance at certain times?" Well, the truth is, asthma is a bit of a mysterious character. It doesn't follow a strict timetable or age preference. Various factors come into play, such as genetics, environmental exposures, and individual health conditions.

Wrapping Up:

In the grand narrative of life, asthma can be an unexpected subplot. It doesn't discriminate based on age, and its timing is often unpredictable. Whether it makes an appearance in the early years, during the school-age adventures, or in the seasoned chapters of life, the key is awareness and action.

If you suspect asthma or notice any symptoms in yourself or your loved ones, don't hesitate to seek medical advice. Early detection and proper management can significantly improve the quality of life for individuals living with asthma.

5.Unmasking the Culprits - What Causes Asthma?

Imagine your body as a finely tuned orchestra, with each part playing a unique role in harmony. Now, imagine that harmony disrupted by an unexpected intruder - asthma. But where does this uninvited guest come from, and why does it choose to visit some of us? Let's unravel the mystery behind the curtain and discover what causes asthma.

The Asthma Enigma:

Asthma, in its essence, is like a puzzle. It involves the airways, those tubes that allow us to breathe, and how they react to certain triggers. But what are these triggers, and why do they send our airways into a frenzy?

A Symphony of Triggers:

- **Genetic Harmony (or Discord):** Like passing down the family recipe for grandma's cookies, asthma can sometimes run in families. If your parents or siblings have asthma, you might be more likely to join the wheezy club. But, and this is important, having a family history doesn't guarantee you'll develop asthma. It just means the odds might be a bit different for you.
- **The Environmental Orchestra:** Imagine the world around you as a vast orchestra, playing tunes that your body reacts to. Common triggers include:
    - **Allergens:** These are tiny troublemakers like pollen, mold spores, pet dander, and dust mites. Your immune system might see them as invaders, triggering the asthma show.
    - **Irritants:** Just as a scratchy tag in your shirt can be annoying, certain things in the air can irritate your airways. Smoke, strong odors, and air pollution can play this role.
- **Respiratory Infections - The Unwanted Soloist:** Sometimes, a cold or respiratory infection can be like that unexpected solo in the middle of a symphony. It can trigger asthma symptoms or make existing symptoms worse. The body's immune response can cause the airways to tighten and become more sensitive.
- **Physical Activity - The Playful Dancer:** Exercise is usually a good thing, but for some with asthma, it can be like a lively dancer disrupting the

calm. Exercise-induced asthma is a real phenomenon, causing shortness of breath, coughing, and wheezing during or after physical activity.

- **Emotional Rollercoaster - The Mood Maestro:** Believe it or not, strong emotions can sometimes play a role in the asthma drama. Stress, excitement, or even laughter can lead to symptoms for some people. It's like the body's way of expressing itself when the emotions take center stage.

The Trigger-Happy Immune System:

Now, let's talk about the immune system, the guardian of our health. In asthma, the immune system can be a bit trigger-happy. It sees harmless things like pollen or pet hair as threats and decides to launch a defense mission. This defense involves releasing chemicals that lead to inflammation and airway tightening - the core elements of an asthma episode.

The Allergic Allure:

For many with asthma, allergies are like the charming but troublesome guest at a party. Allergic reactions can trigger asthma symptoms, creating a tag-team of respiratory challenges. But not everyone with asthma has allergies, and vice versa. They can be separate characters in the asthma story, or they can join forces for a more challenging plotline.

Timing is Everything:

Asthma, much like a theatrical performance, has its own timing. Some people may experience symptoms only in certain seasons, while others may find that specific activities or environments set the stage for asthma to make its entrance.

Putting It All Together:

In the grand production of asthma, it's crucial to understand that it's often a combination of factors at play. Your genetic makeup, the environment you live in, and your body's unique responses all contribute to the storyline. Think of asthma triggers as actors on a stage, each playing a role in the unfolding drama of respiratory challenges.

Conclusion:

In conclusion, what causes asthma is a multifaceted tale. It's not a simple case of one cause fits all. Instead, it's a blend of genetics, environmental factors, immune responses, and sometimes, a dash of unpredictability. The key is to identify your triggers and work on managing them, allowing you to regain control of your respiratory symphony.

6.Navigating the Journey - Is Asthma a Chronic Disease?

Welcome back, dear readers, to our exploration of the asthma landscape. Today, we're diving into a term you might have come across: chronic disease. Is asthma a chronic condition, you ask? Let's untangle the threads of this question and discover what it means for those living with asthma.

The Chronic Conundrum:

First things first, what does "chronic" even mean in the context of health? Think of it like a persistent companion - a condition that likes to linger rather than making a swift exit. A chronic disease isn't your fleeting cold; it's more like a long-term tenant in the house of your well-being.

Asthma Unveiled:

So, is asthma in it for the long haul? The short answer: yes. Asthma is indeed considered a chronic disease. But fear not; being labeled as chronic doesn't mean a life sentence of constant struggles. Let's break it down.

The Persistent Player:

Asthma has a knack for sticking around. Unlike a passing storm, asthma doesn't just blow through and leave everything untouched. It hangs around, affecting the airways and occasionally stirring up a bit of a commotion. But here's the thing: the intensity of this commotion can vary.

Peaks and Valleys:

Asthma is a bit like a rollercoaster, with its ups and downs. Some days, you might hardly notice it - the airways are calm, and breathing is a breeze. Other days, you might find yourself grappling with symptoms like coughing, wheezing, or shortness of breath. It's a journey with peaks and valleys, and managing asthma involves learning how to navigate the terrain.

The Role of Triggers:

Remember those triggers we talked about earlier? They're like mischievous characters in the asthma drama. While asthma itself is chronic, certain triggers can stir the pot and bring symptoms to the forefront. Identifying and managing these triggers is a key part of keeping the chronic nature of asthma in check.

Treatment as a Guide:
Now, let's talk about managing this persistent companion. Just because asthma is chronic doesn't mean you're left to fend for yourself. There's a whole arsenal of tools and strategies to help you steer the course. Inhalers, medications, and lifestyle adjustments become your trusty companions on this journey.

The Importance of Consistency:
Managing chronic conditions, including asthma, often involves a consistent approach. It's not about tackling it head-on when it flares up but rather maintaining a steady routine to keep symptoms at bay. This might mean taking medications as prescribed, keeping an eye on triggers, and working closely with healthcare professionals to adjust your management plan as needed.

Quality of Life Matters:
Here's a crucial point: being labeled as chronic doesn't mean a diminished quality of life. With proper management, many individuals with asthma lead vibrant, active lives. It's about understanding your unique asthma story, recognizing the signs when it whispers, and taking proactive steps to keep it from shouting.

Asthma Across the Lifespan:
Asthma doesn't play favorites when it comes to age. Whether you're a sprightly youngster or enjoying the golden years, asthma can be a part of your life story. The key is adapting your management plan to suit the changing chapters of life.

Wrapping Up:
In the grand narrative of health, asthma is a chapter that unfolds over time. It's a chronic companion, but with the right knowledge and tools, you can learn to coexist and even thrive. So, is asthma a chronic disease? Yes, indeed. But remember, you're the author of your own story, and asthma is just one character in the tale of your well-being.

7.Will It Get Worse With Age?

Greetings, fellow travelers on the asthma journey! As we weave through the chapters of this book, one question might be lingering in the corners of your mind: what about the road ahead? Specifically, is there a risk that your asthma might decide to change its tune as the years roll by? Let's embark on a quest to unravel the mysteries of aging and asthma.

The Symphony of Life:

Life is a grand symphony, and each passing year adds new notes to the composition. But how does asthma fit into this musical journey? Is it a melody that becomes more harmonious with time, or does it introduce unexpected twists and turns?

The Age-Old Question:

First things first, aging is a natural part of life. As the candles on your birthday cake multiply, so do the experiences and changes in your body. But what about asthma? Does it age like fine wine, or does it, like a mischievous sprite, decide to stir up trouble?

The Varied Verses of Asthma:

Asthma is a bit like a chameleon; it can wear different colors in different stages of life. For some, the energetic days of youth might be peppered with occasional asthma whispers. Others might find that as the years add up, so do the challenges of managing asthma.

The Childhood Cadence:

In the early chapters of life, asthma can be like a fleeting guest. Children might experience symptoms that come and go, often triggered by colds, allergies, or vigorous play. But here's the comforting news: many children with asthma find that their symptoms improve as they grow older.

The Adolescent Crescendo:

Ah, adolescence—a time of growth spurts, newfound independence, and, for some, a shift in the asthma melody. Some individuals may find that adolescence brings changes in their asthma symptoms. Hormones and lifestyle factors can influence the respiratory score, adding a layer of complexity to the tune.

The Adult Harmony:

As adulthood unfolds, asthma can play different roles for different individuals. Some may experience a sort of asthma stability, with symptoms remaining relatively consistent. Others might find that the demands of adulthood—work, family, and the general hustle and bustle—add new dynamics to the asthma storyline.

The Golden Years Duet:

And then comes the golden era. As we gracefully age, asthma can continue to be a companion. For some, the challenges of managing asthma might intensify. It's like a gentle reminder that, even in the later chapters of life, staying attuned to asthma's nuances is crucial.

Why the Change in Tune?

Now, you might be wondering, why does asthma decide to switch up its melody? Well, the answer lies in the intricate dance between aging, lifestyle, and the individual's unique asthma script.

- **Changes in the Body Orchestra:** As we age, the body undergoes various changes. Lung function might decrease slightly, and the immune system may evolve. These natural shifts can influence how asthma behaves.
- **Lifestyle Choreography:** The way we live our lives—the choices we make, the environments we inhabit—can impact asthma. Exposure to new triggers, stress, and changes in physical activity levels can all play a role in the evolving asthma narrative.
- **Adherence to the Asthma Score:** Just like a musician following a musical score, adherence to asthma management strategies becomes crucial. Sometimes, the challenges arise not from aging itself but from adjustments needed in how asthma is managed.

The Silver Lining:

Now, for the silver lining—aging doesn't guarantee a worsening of asthma. Many individuals with asthma find that with consistent management, they can continue to lead vibrant, active lives regardless of their age. It's about adapting the score as needed, understanding the rhythm of your own asthma journey.

The Maestro's Advice:

As we conclude this chapter, consider this wisdom from the asthma maestro: pay attention to the notes, embrace the changes in the melody, and conduct your own symphony of well-being. If you ever feel that the tune is taking an unexpected turn, don't hesitate to reach out to your healthcare team for guidance.

Chapter 2

Causes of Asthma & Trigger Factors

Answers following Questions:
What causes asthma?
What causes asthma symptoms or an asthma attack?
What are asthma triggers?
What are the main asthma triggers?
What chemicals, irritants or other substances trigger asthma?
Can medications trigger asthma?
Can weather changes trigger asthma?
Can infections trigger asthma?
Can an allergic reaction trigger asthma?
Is asthma a psychological (psychosomatic) disease?
Why is it sometimes so hard to know what triggers an asthma attack?
Why does my asthma get worse when I am upset or worried about something?
Can I really get asthma symptoms from a plastic Christmas tree?

1. Unraveling the Mystery of Asthma: Understanding Causes, Symptoms, and Triggers

In the grand theater of our bodies, the respiratory system takes center stage. It's a delicate dance of inhales and exhales, an intricate symphony of oxygen and life. But for some, this dance becomes a bit more complicated, a bit more challenging. Welcome to the world of asthma.

The Intricate Web of Asthma Causes:

Imagine your airways as the roadways of a bustling city. Now, picture these roads being guarded by vigilant sentinels, ensuring smooth traffic flow. In a perfect world, this system operates seamlessly, but asthma adds a plot twist to this tale. Asthma is often considered a complex interplay of genetic and environmental factors. It's like a puzzle, and each piece contributes to the overall picture. While some folks are born with a genetic predisposition to asthma, others may develop it due to exposure to certain environmental factors.

Genetics: The Family Blueprint:

In the genetic realm, asthma tends to run in families. If Uncle Joe or Cousin Emily had it, you might find yourself more susceptible. But genetics is just the foundation; it doesn't seal your fate. Think of it as having a family history of loving the arts – it might influence you, but you can still choose to be an accountant if that's your passion.

So, if asthma has a tendency to knock on your family's door, it's like having a heads-up about potential guests. Your body might be more prone to react, but it doesn't mean you can't manage the situation effectively.

Environmental Triggers: The Plot Thickens:

Now, let's dive into the world outside your genes, where environmental triggers are the supporting actors in the asthma drama.

1. Allergens - The Sneaky Culprits:

Allergens are like mischievous characters, triggering the immune system into unnecessary battles. Dust mites, pollen, pet dander – these seemingly harmless elements can become villains in the asthma tale. They infiltrate your airways, setting off alarms and causing a commotion.

Picture your immune system as a diligent guard. It's supposed to discern friend from foe. However, in asthma, this guard can be a bit overzealous, misidentifying a benign speck of dust as a dangerous intruder. This mistaken identity sparks a response, leading to the classic asthma symptoms we know too well.

2. Respiratory Infections - The Uninvited Guests:

Just as your city might face unexpected traffic jams, your respiratory system can encounter uninvited guests in the form of infections. The common cold and flu, for instance, can turn your airways into chaotic thoroughfares, triggering asthma symptoms.

Infections create a perfect storm, making your airways more sensitive and prone to inflammation. It's like the difference between driving on a smooth road versus navigating a pothole-riddled street. When your airways become the latter, asthma symptoms are more likely to make an appearance.

3. Irritants - The Trouble-Makers:

Irritants are the trouble-makers in the asthma storyline. They can be like that annoying neighbor who insists on playing loud music late into the night. Smoke, air pollution, strong odors – these irritants can stir up trouble in your airways.

Imagine your airways as serene gardens. Irritants are the weeds that, when present, can turn this peaceful landscape into a chaotic battleground. They provoke inflammation, making it harder for air to flow smoothly, and cue the entrance of asthma symptoms.

4. Physical Activity - The Unexpected Twist:

Exercise is undoubtedly a hero in the health narrative, but for some with asthma, it can bring an unexpected twist. Exercise-induced bronchoconstriction, also known as exercise-induced asthma, is like a plot twist in the asthma tale.

When you engage in physical activity, your breathing rate increases. For those with asthma, this heightened activity can trigger symptoms. It's not that exercise is the villain; it's more like the hero facing a bit of adversity. With proper management and precautions, individuals with asthma can still embrace the benefits of an active lifestyle.

A Symphony of Symptoms and Triggers:

Now that we've peeked behind the curtain of asthma causes, let's delve into the main act – the symptoms and triggers.

Symphony of Symptoms:

The symptoms of asthma can be likened to the orchestra playing an unexpected tune. Each instrument (or symptom) has its part to play, creating a unique melody of discomfort.

- **Shortness of Breath - The Breathless Note:**

Shortness of breath is like a subtle melody in the background, a persistent reminder that the respiratory performance isn't as smooth as it should be. It's as if the orchestra is missing a beat, leaving you feeling breathless and out of sync.

- **Coughing - The Persistent Drumbeat:**

Coughing is the persistent drumbeat, echoing through the airways. It's the body's way of trying to clear the stage, removing any potential irritants or blockages. Unfortunately, this drumbeat can become disruptive, signaling an asthma episode.

- **Wheezing - The Whistling Flute:**

Wheezing is like the whistling flute, a high-pitched sound signaling the narrowing of airways. It's as if the orchestra has introduced an unexpected instrument, drawing attention to the struggle within.

- **Chest Tightness - The Constricting Strings:**

Chest tightness is akin to the constricting strings in the orchestra. It's a sensation of pressure, as if an invisible force is tightening around your chest. This discomfort is a common player in the asthma symphony.

Triggers: The Plot Unfolds:

Now, let's explore the triggers that can turn the asthma symphony into a crescendo of symptoms.

- **Allergens - The Puppet Masters:**

Allergens take center stage as puppet masters, pulling the strings to provoke an immune response. They can initiate the asthma symphony, prompting symptoms like coughing, wheezing, and shortness of breath.

- **Infections - The Chaotic Ensemble:**

Respiratory infections join the ensemble, creating chaos within the airways. The orchestra becomes disarrayed, with increased mucus production and inflammation contributing to asthma symptoms.

- **Irritants - The Agitators:**

  Irritants act as agitators, disrupting the calm in your respiratory garden. Smoke, pollution, and strong odors can trigger inflammation, leading to a flurry of asthma symptoms.

- **Physical Activity - The Unscripted Scene:**

  Physical activity adds an unscripted scene to the asthma drama. While exercise is generally beneficial, for some, it can become a trigger, inducing symptoms like coughing and shortness of breath.

Understanding the intricate dance of causes, symptoms, and triggers in the asthma narrative allows individuals and their caregivers to better navigate this complex terrain. Armed with knowledge, managing asthma becomes a collaborative effort, where the conductor (you) guides the orchestra toward a harmonious and symptom-free performance.

2. Navigating Asthma Triggers: Medications, Weather, Infections, and Allergic Reactions

In the intricate tapestry of asthma, triggers can be like mischievous sprites, stirring up trouble in the respiratory realm. In this chapter, let's embark on a journey to demystify some common triggers – medications, weather changes, infections, and allergic reactions.

Medications: The Double-Edged Sword

Imagine your body as a finely tuned orchestra, each system playing its part in harmony. Now, think of medications as the conductors, guiding the symphony of your health. While medications are often the heroes in the story, certain ones can be a bit mischievous, especially for those with asthma.

Can Medications Trigger Asthma?

Yes, they can, but not all medications are created equal. Some may be like the virtuoso violinist, enhancing the melody of your health, while others might be the unruly percussionist, causing a bit of chaos.

Nonsteroidal Anti-Inflammatory Drugs (NSAIDs): The Percussion Pitfall

In the world of medications, NSAIDs are like the drummers in our orchestra. While they might be fantastic for addressing pain and inflammation, for some individuals with asthma, they can play a discordant note. Medications like aspirin and ibuprofen can trigger symptoms, leading to coughing, wheezing, or shortness of breath.

Think of it as a drumbeat that goes out of rhythm, disrupting the smooth flow of the respiratory symphony. If you notice any unexpected reactions to these medications, it's crucial to let your healthcare provider know. They can help you find alternative solutions that won't throw your respiratory rhythm off balance.

Beta-Blockers: The Fluctuating Flute

Beta-blockers, often prescribed for conditions like high blood pressure and certain heart conditions, can be like a temperamental flute in our orchestra. While they might be essential for managing other health issues, they can potentially trigger asthma symptoms in some individuals.

These medications work by blocking the effects of adrenaline, which can inadvertently cause the airways to narrow, leading to breathing difficulties. It's like having a flute that decides to play a few unexpected high notes, catching your breath off guard.

Again, communication is key. If you're prescribed beta-blockers and notice any unwelcome changes in your breathing, don't hesitate to share this with your healthcare provider. They can explore alternative medications that won't disrupt the respiratory harmony.

Weather Changes: The Atmospheric Ballet

Weather changes can be like the choreography of the atmosphere, influencing the way we breathe. While we can't control the weather, understanding its role in asthma can help us navigate the atmospheric ballet more effectively.

Can Weather Changes Trigger Asthma?

Yes, they can, and it's like the weather putting on its own performance, complete with twists and turns.

Cold Air: The Brisk Breeze

Cold air can be like a brisk breeze, stirring up trouble for those with asthma. When you breathe in chilly air, your airways might react by narrowing, leading to symptoms like coughing or shortness of breath. It's as if the cold air is playing a prank on your respiratory system, prompting it to tighten up.

To combat this, consider wearing a scarf or a mask over your nose and mouth in cold weather. This simple act can help warm the air before it reaches your lungs, preventing the unexpected cold-induced reactions.

Hot and Humid Weather: The Steamy Symphony

On the other side of the spectrum, hot and humid weather can create its own challenges. The air becomes heavy and laden with moisture, potentially triggering asthma symptoms. It's like the atmosphere deciding to add a bit of humidity to the respiratory symphony, making it a bit harder to breathe.

In humid conditions, staying hydrated is key. Drink plenty of water to keep your airways happy and hydrated. Additionally, if possible, stay indoors during the hottest part of the day to avoid the peak of atmospheric drama.

Thunderstorms: The Atmospheric Showdown

Thunderstorms are like the dramatic showdown in the atmospheric theater. While the rain can clear the air of allergens like pollen, the stormy conditions can also stir up mold spores and other irritants, potentially triggering asthma symptoms.

If you're sensitive to weather changes, it's wise to keep an eye on the forecast. Planning ahead and taking preventive measures, such as using your prescribed medications, can help you weather the storm with minimal respiratory disruption.

Infections: The Unwelcome Intruders

In the grand tale of health, infections can be like unwelcome intruders barging into the respiratory realm. Let's explore how these pesky invaders can influence the asthma narrative.

Can Infections Trigger Asthma?

Yes, they can, and it's like the body's defense system going on high alert. When you're battling an infection, whether it's a cold, flu, or respiratory infection, your immune system kicks into overdrive. While this heightened response is essential for fighting off the invaders, it can also impact your airways.

Respiratory Infections: The Stealthy Saboteurs

Respiratory infections, like the common cold or flu, can be like stealthy saboteurs infiltrating the respiratory orchestra. They create chaos, triggering inflammation and increased mucus production. This can lead to symptoms like coughing, wheezing, and shortness of breath.

It's essential to be vigilant and proactive during cold and flu seasons. Practice good hygiene, such as regular handwashing, to minimize the risk of infections. Additionally, if you have asthma, ensure you're up to date on vaccinations, including the flu shot, to provide an extra layer of protection.

Allergic Reactions: The Immune System's Dilemma

Allergic reactions are like the immune system's dilemma – a case of mistaken identity that can set off a cascade of respiratory reactions. Understanding how allergens play a role in asthma is key to managing these triggers effectively.

Can Allergic Reactions Trigger Asthma?

Yes, they can, and it's like the immune system hitting the panic button unnecessarily. When you encounter allergens, substances that your body mistakenly identifies as harmful, your immune system goes into overdrive. For individuals with asthma, this can lead to the classic symptoms of coughing, wheezing, and difficulty breathing.

Pollen: The Airborne Culprit

Pollen is like the airborne culprit in the allergy drama. When pollen levels are high, especially during spring and fall, it can trigger allergic reactions in some individuals. It's as if the pollen decides to play an unexpected role in the respiratory symphony, leading to a surge in asthma symptoms.

To minimize the impact of pollen, keep an eye on local pollen forecasts. On high pollen days, consider staying indoors as much as possible and keeping windows closed. Using air purifiers with HEPA filters can also help reduce indoor pollen levels.

Dust Mites: The Indoor Intruders

Dust mites are like the unseen intruders in the indoor environment, triggering allergic reactions that can exacerbate asthma. These microscopic creatures thrive in bedding, upholstered furniture, and carpets, making them stealthy but impactful players in the asthma narrative.

To combat dust mites, focus on regular cleaning and dusting. Use allergen-proof covers on pillows and mattresses, and wash bedding in hot water regularly. Creating an environment that's less hospitable to dust mites

3. Unraveling the Mind-Body Connection in Asthma: Beyond the Wheezing

In the intricate tapestry of asthma, the connection between the mind and body is like a delicate dance, each step influencing the other. In this chapter, we'll explore the fascinating interplay between asthma and our emotions, addressing common questions about the psychological aspects of the condition.

Is Asthma a Psychological (Psychosomatic) Disease?

Let's start by debunking a common misconception: asthma is not purely a psychological or psychosomatic disease. While emotions can indeed play a role, asthma has concrete roots in the physiological workings of the respiratory system. It's like a two-sided coin, with both physical and emotional aspects contributing to the overall experience.

Asthma involves inflammation and narrowing of the airways, making it harder to breathe. This isn't a figment of the imagination; it's a tangible response to various triggers, including allergens, infections, and irritants. So, while emotions may influence the course of asthma, they don't single-handedly create the condition.

The Mystery of Asthma Triggers: A Detective Story

Now, let's delve into the enigma of asthma triggers. Why is it sometimes so challenging to pinpoint what sets off an asthma attack?

Why is it Sometimes So Hard to Know What Triggers an Asthma Attack?

Imagine your body as a detective investigating a complex case. Asthma triggers can be like elusive culprits, hiding in plain sight one moment and vanishing the next. The challenge lies in the diversity of triggers and the unique way each person's body responds.

- **Individual Variability:**

  Just as detectives need to adapt their strategies for different cases, asthma triggers vary from person to person. What sets off one individual's asthma might not affect another. This individual variability makes it challenging to create a one-size-fits-all list of triggers.

- **Multiple Culprits at Play:**

  Asthma triggers can be a sneaky bunch, often teaming up to create the perfect storm. It's not uncommon for several factors to contribute to an asthma episode simultaneously. For example, a person might be exposed to a respiratory infection while also facing high levels of air pollution, making it tricky to pinpoint the primary trigger.

- **Delayed Reactions:**

  Like a plot twist in a detective novel, some asthma triggers can have delayed effects. You might encounter a trigger today, but the symptoms might not manifest until tomorrow or the day after. This delayed response can make it challenging to connect the dots between exposure and symptoms.

- **Subtle Environmental Factors:**

  Asthma triggers aren't always obvious villains; sometimes, they're more like background characters in the story. Subtle changes in temperature, humidity, or air quality can impact your respiratory health without a clear culprit standing out.

The key to cracking the case of asthma triggers is diligent observation. Keep a journal to track your activities, surroundings, and emotions when asthma symptoms occur. Over time, patterns may emerge, helping you and your healthcare team identify and manage specific triggers more effectively.

The Mind-Body Connection: Why Does My Asthma Get Worse When I Am Upset or Worried?

Now, let's explore the intricate relationship between emotions and asthma. Why does asthma sometimes seem to tighten its grip when we're upset or worried?

The Stress-Response System:

When you're stressed, worried, or upset, your body activates its stress-response system. Think of it as sounding the alarm in the face of a perceived threat – your body prepares to fight or flee. This response involves the release of stress hormones like adrenaline, which can have physiological effects on various systems, including the respiratory system.

Increased Sensitivity:
Stress can make your airways more sensitive, like turning up the volume on a finely tuned instrument. This heightened sensitivity can make you more susceptible to asthma triggers, even those that might not normally cause symptoms.

Changes in Breathing Patterns:
Emotional distress can also influence your breathing patterns. You might unconsciously start breathing more rapidly or shallowly, which can trigger or exacerbate asthma symptoms. It's like the rhythm of your breath becoming discordant with the harmony your respiratory system usually maintains.

Impact on the Immune System:
Stress has a way of influencing the immune system, potentially making your body more reactive to allergens and irritants. This heightened immune response can contribute to inflammation in the airways, worsening asthma symptoms.

Breaking the Cycle:
The relationship between emotions and asthma is a two-way street. While stress can exacerbate asthma symptoms, the experience of having asthma itself can be stressful. It's a feedback loop that, once established, can be challenging to break. Breaking the cycle involves not only managing stress but also addressing the emotional aspects of living with asthma. Incorporating stress-reduction techniques, such as deep breathing exercises, meditation, or engaging in activities you enjoy, can be valuable tools in your asthma management toolkit.

Anxiety and Asthma: A Tangled Web:
Anxiety, a persistent feeling of unease or worry, can weave a tangled web with asthma. Individuals with asthma may experience anxiety about their health, future asthma attacks, or the impact of the condition on their daily lives. This anxiety, in turn, can contribute to a heightened state of alertness and physiological changes that may worsen asthma symptoms.

It's essential to recognize the interconnected nature of emotions and asthma and address both aspects in your asthma management plan. Working with your healthcare team to develop strategies for stress management and emotional well-being can empower you to navigate the mind-body connection with greater resilience.

In summary, while asthma has concrete physiological roots, the mind and body are intricately connected in the asthma narrative. Understanding the interplay between emotions and asthma triggers allows individuals and caregivers to approach asthma management with a holistic perspective, fostering not only physical well-being but also emotional resilience in the face of this respiratory journey.

Chapter 3

Asthma Symptoms

Answers following Questions:
What does asthma feel like?
What happens during an asthma attack?
What causes an asthma attack?
What are the signs of a severe and dangerous asthma attack?
Can a person die from asthma?
Why do I lose my breath?
How do I know if I am having an asthma attack?
Can the peak flow meter tell me if I need to see the doctor?
Can asthma medication help prevent asthma symptoms?

1.Decoding the Asthma Attack Experience: A Rollercoaster of Breath

In the realm of respiratory health, asthma isn't just a word; it's an experience, a journey that unfolds within the intricate chambers of the lungs. In this chapter, let's embark on a guided tour into the world of asthma, exploring what it feels like, the dynamics of an asthma attack, and the triggers that can set this respiratory rollercoaster into motion.

What Does Asthma Feel Like?

Imagine your lungs as flexible balloons, expanding and contracting with each breath, orchestrating the symphony of life. Now, envision asthma as a gentle disruptor of this rhythm, introducing a set of sensations that can vary from person to person. Let's explore what asthma feels like in the context of the respiratory adventure.

- **The Breathless Ballet:**

  At the heart of the asthma experience is a dance with breathlessness. It's like waltzing through a routine where the steps are harder to execute. As the airways narrow, breathing becomes a delicate balance, and each inhalation feels like a negotiation with the respiratory symphony.

- **The Persistent Cough:**

  Asthma often brings along a persistent cough, like a background percussion instrument in the respiratory orchestra. It's not just any cough; it's the kind that lingers, signaling that the airways might be irritated or constricted.

- **The Whistling Symphony:**

  Wheezing, a high-pitched whistling sound during breathing, can be another element of the asthma melody. It's like the presence of an unexpected instrument, drawing attention to the struggle within the airways. Wheezing isn't always present, but when it joins the symphony, it adds a distinctive note to the respiratory composition.

- **Chest Tightness:**

  Picture a gentle hug that turns into a constricting embrace. That's how individuals with asthma often describe chest tightness. It's a sensation of pressure, as if an invisible force is tightening around the chest, making breathing feel like a constrained endeavor.

- **The Unpredictable Nature:**

  Asthma doesn't always follow a script; it's more like an improvisational jazz performance. Symptoms can come and go, varying in intensity and duration. Some days, breathing may feel effortless, while on others, it's like navigating through an airway obstacle course.

Understanding what asthma feels like is a crucial step in the journey toward effective management. It allows individuals and caregivers to recognize the nuances of the respiratory symphony, paving the way for informed decisions and timely interventions.

What Happens During an Asthma Attack?

An asthma attack is like a sudden storm in the respiratory landscape, disrupting the usual flow of breath and introducing a sense of urgency. Let's unravel the dynamics of an asthma attack, step by step.

- **The Prelude:**

  An asthma attack often begins with a sense of unease – a subtle shift in the respiratory atmosphere. This prelude may involve the gradual onset of symptoms like coughing, wheezing, or shortness of breath. It's like the calm before the storm, signaling that the respiratory symphony is about to take an unexpected turn.

- **The Crescendo:**

  As the attack progresses, symptoms intensify. Breathing becomes more challenging, and the rhythm of the respiratory symphony becomes erratic. Wheezing may become more pronounced, and chest tightness can escalate, creating a crescendo of respiratory distress.

- **The Climax:**

  The climax of an asthma attack is marked by a peak in symptom severity. It's like reaching the top of a rollercoaster, where the challenges are at their zenith. During this phase, individuals may experience significant difficulty in breathing, and the chest tightness can feel particularly pronounced.

- **The Resolution:**

  Fortunately, like the passing of a storm, an asthma attack doesn't last forever. With appropriate interventions, such as using rescue inhalers or seeking medical assistance, the respiratory symphony can gradually return to a more harmonious cadence. The resolution phase involves the easing of symptoms and a gradual return to normal breathing.

Understanding the sequence of an asthma attack empowers individuals and caregivers to respond promptly. Quick action, whether through the use of prescribed medications or seeking medical attention, can often prevent the escalation of symptoms and promote a smoother resolution.

What Causes an Asthma Attack?
The triggers behind an asthma attack are like the invisible puppeteers orchestrating the respiratory drama. Identifying these triggers is crucial in developing an effective asthma management plan. Let's explore some common culprits that can set the stage for an asthma attack.

- **Allergens:**

  Allergens are like mischievous intruders, provoking the immune system into unnecessary battles. Common allergens include pollen, pet dander, dust mites, and mold spores. When these intruders infiltrate the airways, the immune response can lead to inflammation and trigger an asthma attack.

- **Respiratory Infections:**

  Picture a stealthy invasion of respiratory invaders, such as the common cold or flu. Respiratory infections can create chaos in the airways, making them more sensitive and prone to inflammation. This heightened reactivity can contribute to the onset of an asthma attack.

- **Irritants:**

  Asthma triggers can be like trouble-making agitators. Environmental irritants, including smoke, air pollution, and strong odors, can provoke inflammation in the airways, acting as catalysts for asthma attacks. It's like the respiratory system responding to an unwelcome disturbance.

- **Physical Activity:**

  While exercise is generally beneficial, for some individuals with asthma, it can act as a trigger. Exercise-induced bronchoconstriction, commonly known as exercise-induced asthma, involves the narrowing of airways during physical activity. This can lead to symptoms like coughing and shortness of breath, contributing to the occurrence of an asthma attack.

- **Weather Changes:**

  Weather can be like the atmospheric choreographer, influencing the respiratory performance. Cold air, hot and humid conditions, and thunderstorms are examples of weather-related triggers. These changes in atmospheric conditions can impact airway sensitivity and contribute to the onset of asthma attacks.

- **Emotional Factors:**

  Emotions, such as stress and anxiety, can influence the respiratory symphony. When individuals are upset or worried, the stress-response system activates, potentially making the airways more sensitive. Emotional distress can contribute to changes in breathing patterns, exacerbating asthma symptoms and increasing the likelihood of an asthma attack.

Recognizing the diverse cast of asthma triggers is essential for effective asthma management. By identifying and minimizing exposure to these triggers, individuals and caregivers can play an active role in reducing the frequency and severity of asthma attacks.

In conclusion, asthma is not just a diagnosis; it's an intricate journey that involves understanding the sensations, dynamics, and triggers that shape the respiratory experience. By unraveling the mysteries of asthma, individuals and caregivers can navigate this respiratory adventure with greater awareness, resilience, and the tools needed for effective management.

2.What Are the Signs of a Severe and Dangerous Asthma Attack?

Recognizing the signs of a severe asthma attack is akin to being the captain of a ship, navigating through stormy waters with a keen eye for danger. While asthma attacks can vary in intensity, certain signs indicate that immediate action is needed.

- **Extreme Shortness of Breath:**

  If you find yourself struggling for breath, gasping for air, and unable to speak in full sentences, it's a red flag. Extreme shortness of breath suggests that the airways are significantly narrowed, and urgent intervention is necessary.

- **Inability to Speak or Eat:**

  When an asthma attack reaches a critical point, individuals may find it difficult to speak or eat. This is a sign that the respiratory distress is severe, and immediate medical attention is crucial.

- **Bluish Lips or Fingernails (Cyanosis):**

  Cyanosis is a serious sign that indicates a lack of oxygen in the bloodstream. If the lips or fingernails turn bluish, it suggests a severe oxygen deficiency and demands prompt medical assistance.

- **Use of Muscles Between Ribs (Retractions):**

  During a severe asthma attack, the body may employ extra effort to breathe. This can result in the use of muscles between the ribs (retractions), indicating that the respiratory distress has escalated.

- **Increased Heart Rate:**

  An elevated heart rate, especially when combined with other severe symptoms, can be a warning sign of a dangerous asthma attack. It indicates that the body is under considerable stress, and urgent medical attention is needed.

- **Limited Improvement with Rescue Inhaler:**

  If the usual rescue inhaler provides limited relief or if symptoms return shortly after using it, it suggests that the asthma attack is severe, and professional medical assistance is imperative.

Can a Person Die from Asthma?

The prospect of a life-threatening asthma attack can be frightening, but it's essential to approach this question with a balanced perspective. While asthma is a serious condition that requires diligent management, most individuals can effectively control their symptoms with proper treatment and adherence to an asthma action plan.

However, in rare cases, severe asthma attacks can lead to a life-threatening situation called status asthmaticus. This is an extreme and prolonged asthma attack that doesn't respond well to standard treatments. It requires immediate emergency medical attention.

The key to preventing life-threatening situations is proactive asthma management. Individuals and caregivers should work closely with healthcare providers to develop a comprehensive asthma action plan. This plan should include:

- **Regular Medication Management:**

  Adhering to prescribed medications, including controller and rescue medications, is crucial for maintaining optimal asthma control.

- **Identifying and Avoiding Triggers:**

  Recognizing and minimizing exposure to asthma triggers, such as allergens and irritants, can significantly reduce the risk of severe attacks.

- **Regular Monitoring and Check-ups:**

  Regular check-ups with healthcare providers and ongoing monitoring of asthma symptoms help identify potential issues early on, allowing for timely intervention.

- **Emergency Action Plan:**

  Having a clear and actionable emergency plan is vital. This plan should outline steps to take in the event of worsening symptoms and provide guidance on when to seek emergency medical assistance.

By staying proactive and informed, individuals and caregivers can effectively manage asthma and reduce the risk of life-threatening situations.

Why Do I Lose My Breath?

The sensation of losing one's breath during an asthma attack is like being caught in a moment where the air becomes elusive, slipping through your grasp. Understanding this sensation involves unraveling the intricate dance between the respiratory system and the triggers that can disrupt its harmony.

- **Airway Constriction:**

  One of the primary reasons for the sensation of losing breath in asthma is the constriction of the airways. During an asthma attack, the muscles surrounding the airways tighten, narrowing the passages through which air flows. This constriction makes it challenging for air to move freely, leading to the sensation of breathlessness.

- **Inflammation:**

  Inflammation plays a pivotal role in asthma, contributing to the swelling of the airway walls. As the airways become inflamed, the space available for airflow decreases. This inflammation, combined with the tightening of muscles, creates a sense of resistance, making each breath feel more effortful.

- **Increased Mucus Production:**

  The respiratory system responds to triggers by producing excess mucus, intended to trap and remove irritants. However, during an asthma attack, this response can backfire. The excess mucus can further obstruct the already narrowed airways, contributing to the feeling of breathlessness.

- **Changes in Breathing Patterns:**

  The body's natural response to the perception of restricted airflow is to alter breathing patterns. Individuals may unconsciously start breathing more rapidly or shallowly, exacerbating the sensation of breathlessness. These changes in breathing patterns are part of the body's attempt to cope with the challenges imposed by constricted airways.

- **Oxygen Deficiency:**

  As the airways narrow and breathing becomes more difficult, the body may experience a decrease in oxygen levels. This can lead to a sensation of breathlessness, as the body signals the need for more oxygen.

Understanding the mechanics behind the sensation of losing breath is a crucial step in effective asthma management. It empowers individuals and caregivers to recognize the early signs of worsening symptoms and take prompt action, whether through the use of rescue medications or seeking medical assistance.

In conclusion, navigating the storm of asthma attacks involves understanding the triggers, recognizing the signs of severe episodes, addressing concerns about potential dangers, and unraveling the sensation of losing breath. By approaching asthma management with knowledge and proactive measures, individuals and caregivers can empower themselves to navigate the respiratory journey with resilience and confidence.

3.A Breath of Clarity: Recognizing an Asthma Attack and the Role of the Peak Flow Meter

In the journey of managing asthma, being attuned to the signals of an impending asthma attack is like having a compass to navigate the respiratory landscape. In this chapter, we'll explore the common signs that indicate you might be having an asthma attack and shed light on the role of a simple yet powerful tool – the peak flow meter – in helping you gauge when it's time to seek medical guidance.

How Do I Know If I Am Having an Asthma Attack?

Imagine your body as a well-tuned instrument, playing the symphony of breath effortlessly. Now, consider an asthma attack as a moment when the usual melody takes an unexpected turn. Recognizing the signs of an asthma attack involves being in tune with your body and paying attention to subtle cues. Here are common indicators that you might be experiencing an asthma attack:

- **Shortness of Breath:**

  Feeling unusually short of breath, as if you can't get enough air, is a hallmark sign of an asthma attack. It's like a sudden shift in the rhythm of your breath, prompting you to pay attention to the change.

- **Persistent Cough:**

  If you find yourself coughing persistently, especially if the cough is accompanied by wheezing or a whistling sound, it could be a sign that your airways are constricted. This is like a warning note in the respiratory symphony, signaling potential trouble.

- **Chest Tightness:**

  Chest tightness can feel like an invisible hand squeezing your chest. It's a sensation of pressure that accompanies an asthma attack, making each breath feel constrained. If you notice an unusual tightness in your chest, it's time to consider the possibility of an asthma episode.

- **Wheezing Sounds:**

  Wheezing, a high-pitched whistling sound when breathing, is often associated with asthma. If you hear these unexpected notes in your breath, especially during exhalation, it's a signal that your airways may be narrowed, and an asthma attack could be underway.

- **Difficulty Speaking or Completing Sentences:**

  During an asthma attack, you might find it challenging to speak in full sentences or express yourself verbally. This difficulty in articulating words is a sign that your breathing is compromised and warrants attention.

- **Increased Respiratory Rate:**

  If you notice a sudden increase in your breathing rate, characterized by rapid and shallow breaths, it could indicate respiratory distress. This change in breathing pattern is your body's way of responding to the challenges posed by constricted airways.

- **Use of Accessory Muscles:**

  In severe cases, you might observe the use of accessory muscles during breathing. These muscles, located between the ribs and in the neck, are not typically engaged during normal breathing. If you notice these muscles coming into play, it's a sign that your respiratory system is under strain.

- **Anxiety or Agitation:**

  Emotional responses, such as heightened anxiety or agitation, can accompany an asthma attack. This is often a result of the body's stress response to the perceived threat of restricted airflow.

Understanding these signs allows you to take proactive steps in managing asthma. If you experience a combination of these symptoms, it's crucial to follow your asthma action plan, which may include using rescue medications, such as an inhaler, and seeking medical assistance if symptoms persist or worsen.

Can the Peak Flow Meter Tell Me If I Need to See the Doctor?

Enter the peak flow meter – a simple device that holds the power to provide valuable insights into your respiratory health. Think of it as a personal gauge, allowing you to measure the force with which you can expel air from your lungs. The peak flow meter is not just a medical tool; it's a companion in your asthma journey, helping you track changes in your lung function and providing early indications of potential issues.

Understanding the Peak Flow Meter:
The peak flow meter is a handheld device with a mouthpiece and a marker that moves along a scale. When you take a deep breath and blow forcefully into the mouthpiece, the marker moves to a position on the scale, indicating your peak expiratory flow (PEF) – essentially, how fast you can breathe out.

How to Use the Peak Flow Meter:
Using the peak flow meter is simple and can be integrated into your daily routine. Here's a step-by-step guide:

- **Stand Up Straight:**

  Stand up straight, ensuring that you have a clear, unobstructed path for airflow.

- **Reset the Marker:**

  If your peak flow meter has a marker, ensure that it is reset to the bottom of the scale.

- **Take a Deep Breath:**

  Take a deep breath and place the mouthpiece in your mouth, forming a tight seal with your lips.

- **Blow Out Forcefully:**

  Blow out as forcefully and quickly as you can into the mouthpiece. Make sure to give it your best effort.

- **Record the Reading:**

  Note the position of the marker on the scale. This number represents your peak expiratory flow.

Interpreting Peak Flow Readings:
The numbers on the peak flow meter scale are categorized into three zones – green, yellow, and red:

- **Green Zone:**

  If your reading falls within the green zone, it indicates that your asthma is well-controlled, and you can continue with your usual management plan.

- **Yellow Zone:**

  A reading in the yellow zone suggests a cautionary phase. It may indicate that your asthma is worsening, and you should follow your asthma action plan, which may involve adjusting medications or seeking medical advice.

- **Red Zone:**

  If your reading falls into the red zone, it signals a potentially serious situation. This indicates a significant decline in lung function, and you should seek immediate medical attention.

Can the Peak Flow Meter Help Determine When to See the Doctor?
Absolutely. The peak flow meter serves as an early-warning system, providing insights into changes in your lung function before you may even feel significant symptoms. Here's how the peak flow meter can guide you in deciding when to see the doctor:

- **Regular Monitoring:**

  By regularly using the peak flow meter, you establish a baseline for your typical lung function. Any deviations from this baseline for your typical lung function. Any deviations from this baseline can be indicative of changes in your asthma.

- **Identifying Trends:**

  Trends in your peak flow readings can reveal patterns of improvement or decline. If you notice a consistent decrease in peak flow readings over several days, it's a sign that your asthma may be worsening.

- **Early Intervention:**

  The peak flow meter allows for early intervention. If your readings enter the yellow zone, it's a signal to follow your asthma action plan and take steps to prevent further deterioration. This may involve adjusting medication doses or seeking medical advice promptly.

- **Red Zone Alert:**

  A reading in the red zone is a clear indication that you should seek immediate medical attention. This level of decline in lung function may require prompt intervention to prevent a severe asthma episode.

Integrating the Peak Flow Meter into Your Asthma Management:
The peak flow meter is not just a diagnostic tool; it's a proactive measure that empowers you to take charge of your asthma. Here are some tips for integrating the peak flow meter into your asthma management routine:

- **Consistency is Key:**

  Aim for consistency in the timing of your peak flow measurements. Whether it's in the morning, evening, or both, establishing a routine helps in tracking changes effectively.

- **Record Keeping:**

  Keep a record of your peak flow readings. This can be in the form of a simple chart or a diary. Regular record-keeping helps you and your healthcare provider identify patterns and make informed decisions.

- **Communication with Healthcare Providers:**

  Share your peak flow readings with your healthcare provider during check-ups. This information provides valuable insights into the effectiveness of your current asthma management plan and allows for adjustments as needed.

- **Educate Caregivers:**

  If you're a caregiver for someone with asthma, familiarize yourself with the peak flow meter. Understanding how to use and interpret the peak flow meter readings enables you to provide valuable support to your loved one.

- **Regular Maintenance:**

Ensure that your peak flow meter is in good working condition. Regularly check for any damage or wear and follow the manufacturer's guidelines for cleaning and maintenance.

In conclusion, recognizing the signs of an asthma attack involves being attuned to your body's signals, while the peak flow meter adds an extra layer of clarity to your asthma management. By embracing this simple yet powerful tool, you can navigate your respiratory journey with confidence, using early indicators to take proactive steps in maintaining optimal lung function and seeking medical advice when needed. The peak flow meter is not just a device; it's a partner in your quest for respiratory well-being.

Chapter 4
Asthma Prognosis: Understanding Longevity, Progression & Hope

Answers following Questions:
Can my asthma be cured?
Is there a risk that my asthma will get worse with age?
Can I outgrow my asthma?
Is asthma a life-long disease?
Is it worse getting asthma when you are old?

Unveiling the Asthma Journey: Understanding Longevity, Progression, and Hope

Embarking on the journey of asthma is like navigating an ever-changing landscape, where questions about the future often take center stage. In this chapter, we'll delve into the queries that many individuals with asthma and their caregivers ponder: Can asthma be cured? Does age play a role in the progression of asthma? Can one outgrow asthma? Is asthma a lifelong companion, and does it manifest differently in later years? Let's unravel these threads and gain insights into the nuanced nature of asthma.

Can My Asthma Be Cured?

The desire for a cure is a natural aspiration when faced with a chronic condition like asthma. However, it's essential to approach this question with a realistic perspective. As of now, asthma is considered a chronic condition, meaning that it doesn't have a definitive cure in the conventional sense.

What is achievable, though, is effective management that allows individuals to lead fulfilling lives with minimal impact from asthma. Management strategies typically involve a combination of medications, lifestyle adjustments, and an astute awareness of triggers. By working closely with healthcare providers and adhering to a personalized asthma action plan, many individuals experience significant relief from symptoms and are able to maintain good respiratory health.

It's important to note that asthma is highly variable among individuals. Some may find their symptoms well-controlled with relatively straightforward management, while others may face greater challenges. The emphasis is on achieving optimal control and quality of life rather than seeking an elusive cure.

Is There a Risk That My Asthma Will Get Worse with Age?

Aging is an inevitable part of life, and it's natural to wonder how asthma might evolve over the years. The relationship between asthma and aging is multifaceted, and several factors come into play:

- **Individual Variability:**

  Asthma manifests differently in each individual. While some people experience consistent control or even improvement in symptoms as they age, others may face challenges or an exacerbation of symptoms.

- **Changing Immune Response:**

  As the immune system undergoes changes with age, the inflammatory response in the airways can also be influenced. This variability can contribute to differences in how asthma presents itself over time.

- **Coexisting Health Conditions:**

  Age often brings an increased likelihood of other health conditions. The interplay between asthma and these coexisting conditions can influence the overall trajectory of respiratory health.

- **Hormonal Changes:**

  Hormonal changes, especially in women, can impact asthma symptoms. Some women may experience changes in asthma severity or patterns during hormonal fluctuations, such as during menstruation or menopause.

While there's no universal rule, it's crucial for individuals with asthma to maintain open communication with their healthcare providers as they age. Regular check-ups, adjustments to the asthma management plan, and proactive measures can contribute to sustained respiratory well-being.

Can I Outgrow My Asthma?
The prospect of outgrowing asthma is a hopeful consideration, especially for those who experienced asthma symptoms in childhood. In some cases, particularly with childhood-onset asthma, individuals may indeed see a reduction in the frequency and severity of symptoms as they enter adolescence and adulthood.
Several factors contribute to the possibility of outgrowing asthma:

- **Changes in Airway Structure:**

  As individuals grow, their airways undergo structural changes. This natural development can contribute to an improvement in airway function and a reduction in asthma symptoms.

- **Changing Immune Response:**

- The immune system undergoes maturation as children transition to adulthood. This maturation can result in a decreased reactivity of the airways to triggers, leading to a reduction in asthma symptoms.
- **Environmental Influences:**

  Changes in living environments, exposure to different allergens, and lifestyle modifications can also play a role. For example, moving to an area with fewer asthma triggers or making adjustments to living conditions can positively impact asthma outcomes.

However, it's important to note that not everyone outgrows asthma. The trajectory of asthma varies widely among individuals, and some may continue to experience symptoms into adulthood. Additionally, adult-onset asthma can occur, presenting new challenges for individuals who may not have experienced asthma in their earlier years.

Regular monitoring, adherence to an asthma management plan, and ongoing communication with healthcare providers are crucial, whether individuals experience a reduction in symptoms or continue to manage asthma into adulthood.

Is Asthma a Life-Long Disease?

In the majority of cases, asthma is considered a chronic, lifelong condition. The chronic nature of asthma stems from its underlying characteristics, such as airway inflammation and hyperresponsiveness. While there may not be a cure that eradicates asthma entirely, effective management can significantly mitigate its impact on daily life.

The goal of asthma management is to achieve and maintain optimal control over symptoms, allowing individuals to lead active, fulfilling lives. Management typically involves:

- **Medications:**

  Both controller and rescue medications are prescribed to manage and prevent asthma symptoms. Controller medications work to control inflammation over the long term, while rescue medications provide quick relief during symptom flare-ups.

- **Lifestyle Adjustments:**

  Identifying and minimizing exposure to asthma triggers, maintaining a healthy lifestyle, and avoiding tobacco smoke are integral components of asthma management.

- **Regular Monitoring:**

Periodic check-ups with healthcare providers, regular monitoring of symptoms, and, for some, the use of tools like peak flow meters contribute to effective asthma management.

- **Asthma Action Plan:**

  Developing and adhering to an asthma action plan provides individuals with a clear set of instructions for managing symptoms and knowing when to seek medical assistance.

While asthma may persist throughout life, advancements in medical research and treatment options continue to enhance the quality of life for individuals with asthma. By staying proactive in managing the condition, individuals can minimize the impact of asthma on their daily activities and overall well-being.

Is It Worse Getting Asthma When You Are Old?

The experience of getting asthma later in life can present unique challenges. Asthma that develops in adulthood is often referred to as adult-onset asthma, and its causes and manifestations can differ from childhood-onset asthma.

- **Diagnostic Challenges:**

  Diagnosing asthma in older adults can be challenging due to the overlap of symptoms with other respiratory conditions, such as chronic obstructive pulmonary disease (COPD). This can lead to delays in diagnosis and treatment.

- **Coexisting Health Conditions:**

  Older adults may have a higher prevalence of other health conditions, such as heart disease or arthritis. The presence of these conditions can complicate asthma management and influence treatment choices.

- **Medication Considerations:**

  Older adults may be taking multiple medications for various health conditions. It's crucial for healthcare providers to consider potential interactions and tailor asthma medications accordingly.

- **Reduced Lung Function:**

  Aging is associated with a natural decline in lung function. When asthma is added to the equation, the impact on respiratory health can be more pronounced. This emphasizes the importance of effective asthma management to maintain optimal lung function.

- **Response to Treatment:**

  While asthma is a manageable condition at any age, older adults may experience variations in how their bodies respond to medications. Close monitoring and adjustments to treatment plans may be necessary.

It's important for older adults who develop asthma to seek timely medical attention and collaborate closely with healthcare providers to tailor a management plan that aligns with their unique needs and circumstances. Addressing asthma in later years is about maintaining respiratory.

Chapter 5

Asthma Non-Medical Treatment: Practical Strategies for Managing Asthma Triggers

Answers following Questions:

How can I avoid common triggers?

What can I do to improve my home environment in general?

I'm allergic to pets/furry animals, what can I do?

Should I get a central vacuum cleaner?

I'm allergic to dust mites, what can I do?

Can I reduce my asthma if I get an air purifier?

Can acupuncture help my asthma?

A Breath of Fresh Air: Navigating Asthma-Friendly Environments

In the intricate dance of asthma management, the environment in which you live plays a starring role. This chapter is your guide to creating a haven that supports respiratory health, covering topics from avoiding common triggers to exploring the potential benefits of air purifiers and acupuncture. Let's embark on a journey toward an asthma-friendly environment that fosters well-being and breathes ease into your daily life.

How Can I Avoid Common Triggers?

Imagine your home as a sanctuary, guarded against the triggers that can set off the unwelcome symphony of asthma symptoms. Avoiding common triggers involves creating a shield around you, making your living space a haven of clean air. Here are practical steps to minimize exposure to common triggers:

- **Allergen-Proof Bedding:**

  Invest in allergen-proof pillow and mattress covers to create a barrier against dust mites. Wash bedding regularly in hot water to further reduce allergen levels.

- **Regular Cleaning:**

  Dust and vacuum your home regularly, paying attention to often overlooked areas such as curtains, blinds, and upholstery. Use a vacuum cleaner with a HEPA filter to trap small particles and prevent them from recirculating into the air.

- **Control Humidity:**

  Keep humidity levels in check, as dust mites thrive in humid environments. Use dehumidifiers in damp areas, and consider air conditioning to help maintain a comfortable and dry indoor climate.

- **Pet-Free Zones:**

  If you have furry friends but are allergic to pets, establish designated pet-free zones in your home. Keep pets out of bedrooms, and use high-efficiency air purifiers to help reduce pet dander in the air.

- **Ventilation:**

  Ensure proper ventilation in your home by using exhaust fans in kitchens and bathrooms. Good ventilation helps prevent the buildup of indoor pollutants.

- **Smoke-Free Environment:**

  Avoid smoking indoors, as tobacco smoke is a potent asthma trigger. Establish a smoke-free policy in your home to protect respiratory health.

- **Mind Your Plants:**

  While indoor plants can be aesthetically pleasing, certain molds may thrive in the soil. Be mindful of mold growth and choose plants that are less likely to contribute to indoor allergens.

- **Regular Pest Control:**

  Implement regular pest control measures to minimize the presence of cockroaches and other pests, which can be asthma triggers.

By adopting these measures, you create an environment that is less conducive to common asthma triggers, providing a foundation for better respiratory health.

What Can I Do to Improve My Home Environment in General?
Transforming your home into a respiratory haven involves more than just avoiding triggers; it's about fostering an overall environment that promotes well-being. Consider the following tips to improve your home environment:

- **Optimal Indoor Temperature:**

  Maintain a comfortable indoor temperature, as extremes of heat or cold can trigger asthma symptoms. Use heating and cooling systems to regulate temperature.

- **Natural Light and Ventilation:**

  Maximize natural light and ventilation by opening windows when weather permits. Fresh air and natural light contribute to a positive and invigorating indoor atmosphere.

- **Asthma-Friendly Flooring:**

  Opt for flooring options that are easy to clean and do not trap allergens. Hardwood, tile, or laminate flooring are preferable to carpets, which can harbor dust mites and pet dander.

- **Air Purifiers:**

  Consider using air purifiers equipped with HEPA filters to capture airborne particles. Place them in commonly used areas, especially in bedrooms, for enhanced air quality.

- **Regular Maintenance:**

  Stay on top of home maintenance tasks, such as fixing leaks promptly to prevent mold growth, cleaning air vents, and servicing heating and cooling systems regularly.

- **Reduce Clutter:**

  Minimize clutter, as it provides fewer hiding spots for dust and allergens. Streamlining your living space makes it easier to keep clean and reduces potential triggers.

- **Create a Relaxing Sleep Environment:**

  Pay attention to your sleep environment by choosing hypoallergenic bedding, maintaining a comfortable temperature, and minimizing potential allergens in the bedroom.

- **Incorporate Indoor Plants:**

  Select indoor plants known for their air-purifying qualities, such as snake plants, peace lilies, and spider plants. These plants can help improve indoor air quality.

By incorporating these practices into your home routine, you not only reduce asthma triggers but also create a supportive environment that contributes to overall respiratory wellness.

I'm Allergic to Pets/Furry Animals, What Can I Do?

Being allergic to pets doesn't mean you have to bid farewell to furry companionship. With thoughtful measures, you can enjoy the company of pets while minimizing the impact of allergens. Here's a guide to navigating life with pets when you have allergies:

- **Designate Pet-Free Zones:**

  Create areas in your home where pets are not allowed, especially in bedrooms. This provides a refuge from allergens, allowing you to enjoy a clean and asthma-friendly space.

- **Grooming Routine:**

  Regular grooming of pets is key to managing allergens. Brushing your pet outside can help reduce shedding, and using pet wipes or hypoallergenic shampoos can minimize dander.

- **Wash Bedding Frequently:**

  Wash pet bedding, blankets, and any other fabric that comes into contact with your pets regularly. Using allergen-proof covers for pillows and mattresses can further minimize exposure.

- **HEPA Air Purifiers:**

  Invest in high-efficiency particulate air (HEPA) purifiers to capture pet dander and other airborne particles. Place these purifiers in areas where you and your pets spend the most time.

- **Vacuum with HEPA Filters:**

  Use a vacuum cleaner equipped with a HEPA filter to effectively capture pet dander. Vacuuming regularly, including carpets, rugs, and upholstery, helps maintain a clean environment.

- **Consider Allergy-Friendly Pets:**

  Some pets are considered more hypoallergenic than others. Breeds with hair instead of fur, such as poodles and certain types of terriers, may produce fewer allergens.

- **Regular Veterinary Check-ups:**

  Ensure that your pets receive regular veterinary check-ups to address any skin or coat issues that may contribute to increased allergen levels.

- **Consult with an Allergist:**

  If you're considering bringing a pet into your home and have allergies, consult with an allergist beforehand. They can provide insights into potential allergic reactions and offer personalized advice.

With these strategies, you can enjoy the companionship of pets while maintaining a home environment that is conducive to respiratory health.

Should I Get a Central Vacuum Cleaner?

The choice of a vacuum cleaner can significantly impact indoor air quality, especially for individuals with asthma. A central vacuum cleaner, which differs from traditional portable vacuum cleaners, may offer certain advantages:

- **Improved Filtration:**

  Central vacuum systems often feature enhanced filtration, including HEPA filters. These filters effectively trap smaller particles, preventing them from recirculating into the air during vacuuming.

- **Reduced Allergen Exposure:**

  With a central vacuum system, the motor and dust collection bin are typically located outside the living areas. This can reduce the risk of allergen exposure during the vacuuming process.

- **Less Noise and Vibration:**

  Central vacuum systems are known for being quieter than traditional vacuum cleaners. The reduced noise and vibration can be beneficial for individuals who may be sensitive to the sound and movement of vacuuming.

- **Convenience and Reach:**

  Central vacuum systems often come with long hoses, allowing for extended reach without the need to carry a heavy unit from room to room. This convenience can make vacuuming more accessible.

While central vacuum cleaners offer certain advantages, it's essential to consider individual preferences and needs. Traditional vacuum cleaners with HEPA filters can also be effective in managing asthma triggers, especially if they are well-maintained and used regularly.

I'm Allergic to Dust Mites, What Can I Do?

Dust mites, microscopic creatures that thrive in household dust, are common asthma triggers. Taking steps to minimize exposure to dust mites can significantly improve respiratory health. Here's a roadmap to creating a dust mite-resistant environment:

- **Allergen-Proof Bedding:**

  Encase pillows, mattresses, and box springs in allergen-proof covers to create a barrier against dust mites. Wash bedding regularly in hot water to kill dust mites and remove allergens.

- **Wash Bedding and Linens:**

  Wash bedding, including sheets, pillowcases, and blankets, in hot water at least once a week. Use a water temperature of 130°F (54°C) or higher to effectively eliminate dust mites.

- **Choose Hypoallergenic Pillows and Bedding:**

  Opt for pillows and bedding labeled as hypoallergenic, as they are designed to resist dust mites and allergens.

- **Use Washable Stuffed Toys:**

  If you or your child has stuffed toys, choose washable options. Regularly washing stuffed toys in hot water can help control dust mites.

- **Control Humidity Levels:**

  Maintain indoor humidity levels between 30% and 50% to create an environment less conducive to dust mites. Use dehumidifiers in damp areas if necessary.

- **Vacuum with HEPA Filters:**

  Regularly vacuum carpets, rugs, and upholstery using a vacuum cleaner equipped with a HEPA filter. Vacuuming helps remove dust mites and their waste.

- **Wooden or Tiled Flooring:**

  Consider hardwood, tile, or laminate flooring instead of carpets, as they are easier to clean and less likely to harbor dust mites.

- **Regular Dusting:**

  Dust surfaces in your home regularly using a damp cloth or a microfiber duster. Dry dusting can stir up dust mites, while damp dusting captures them effectively.

By incorporating these practices into your cleaning routine, you create an environment that is less conducive to dust mites, contributing to improved respiratory health.

Can I Reduce My Asthma If I Get an Air Purifier?

The quest for cleaner air is a common consideration for individuals with asthma, and air purifiers can play a role in achieving this goal. Here's a closer look at the potential benefits of air purifiers for asthma management:

- **Particle Removal:**

  Air purifiers equipped with HEPA filters can effectively capture particles such as dust, pollen, pet dander, and mold spores. This particle removal can contribute to better indoor air quality.

- **Reduced Allergen Levels:**

  By capturing and trapping airborne allergens, air purifiers can help reduce the levels of common asthma triggers in the indoor environment.

- **Smoke and Odor Control:**

  Air purifiers with activated carbon filters can help control odors and remove smoke particles from the air. This can be beneficial for individuals with asthma triggered by smoke exposure.

- **Asthma-Friendly Filters:**

  Choose air purifiers with filters specifically designed for asthma management. Look for features such as HEPA filters and activated carbon filters to address a range of airborne pollutants.

- **Improved Indoor Air Quality:**

  Overall, the use of air purifiers contributes to improved indoor air quality. This is particularly important for individuals spending a significant amount of time indoors.

While air purifiers can be a valuable addition to asthma management, it's essential to consider them as part of a comprehensive approach. Other measures, such as regular cleaning, proper ventilation, and allergen reduction strategies, should also be incorporated for optimal respiratory health.

Can Acupuncture Help My Asthma?

The exploration of alternative therapies often leads individuals to consider acupuncture as a potential avenue for asthma management. Acupuncture, an ancient Chinese practice involving the insertion of thin needles into specific points on the body, has been studied for its potential effects on asthma. Here's an overview of the considerations:

- **Holistic Approach:**

  Acupuncture is rooted in a holistic approach to health, aiming to balance the body's energy or qi. Some individuals with asthma explore acupuncture as a complementary therapy to address underlying imbalances.

- **Potential Benefits:**

  While research on acupuncture and asthma is ongoing, some studies suggest that acupuncture may have anti-inflammatory effects and could potentially influence immune system responses. These effects may be relevant to asthma management.

- **Symptom Relief:**

  Some individuals report symptom relief and improved quality of life after undergoing acupuncture. This may include a reduction in the frequency and severity of asthma symptoms.

- **Individual Responses:**

  Responses to acupuncture can vary among individuals. Some may find it beneficial in managing asthma, while others may not experience significant effects. The individualized nature of acupuncture requires consideration of personal responses.

- **Complementary Approach:**

  Acupuncture is often considered as a complementary therapy rather than a standalone treatment for asthma. It is not intended to replace conventional asthma management but may be explored in conjunction with established medical interventions.

- **Consultation with Healthcare Providers:**

  Before incorporating acupuncture into your asthma management plan, consult with your healthcare provider. They can provide guidance on integrating acupuncture into your overall asthma care and help ensure a coordinated approach.

While acupuncture holds promise for some individuals, it's important to approach it with an informed perspective. Work closely with your healthcare team to determine the most effective and personalized strategies for managing your asthma.

In conclusion, crafting an asthma-friendly environment involves a combination of thoughtful choices, strategic measures, and a commitment to respiratory wellness. By navigating common triggers, optimizing your home environment, and exploring complementary approaches, you empower yourself to breathe easier and embrace a lifestyle that supports optimal asthma management.

Chapter 6

Asthma Medical Treatment: Practical Strategies for Managing Asthma

Answers following Questions:
What are controllers?
What are relievers?
What are combination medications?
What effects do anti-inflammatory medications have?
What effects do airway opener medications have?
What are glucocorticosteroids?
Why are glucocorticosteroid medications inhaled?
When and why are corticosteroid tablets or injections used?
What is the difference between a corticosteroid and an anabolic steroid?
What are inhaled non-steroidal anti-inflammatory medications?
Is there an effective alternative to using inhaled corticosteroids?
Do I still need my inhaled corticosteroid if I feel OK?
What anti-inflammatory medication can I take for a strained muscle, aching joints, severe back pain or rheumatism, for example?
What is hyposensitisation (vaccination)?
I'm troubled by my asthma when outdoors in cold weather. What can I do?

*Apologies, this chapter contains Medical terminologies. However, I've tried to make them easy to understand.

Navigating the Medication Maze: A Clear Guide to Asthma Medications

In the realm of asthma management, medications serve as essential tools to control symptoms, provide relief, and enhance overall respiratory well-being. This chapter is your compass through the medication maze, shedding light on controllers, relievers, combination medications, anti-inflammatory wonders, airway openers, and the intriguing world of glucocorticosteroids. Let's embark on a journey to demystify asthma medications and empower you with the knowledge to breathe easy.

1. What Are Controllers?

Controllers are the unsung heroes of asthma management, working behind the scenes to keep symptoms in check and prevent asthma flare-ups. Think of controllers as the steady architects, crafting a foundation of stability for your respiratory health. These medications, typically taken daily, aim to address the underlying inflammation in the airways, reducing the frequency and severity of asthma symptoms.

Common types of controller medications include:

- **Inhaled Corticosteroids (ICS):**

  Inhaled corticosteroids are like the superheroes of anti-inflammatory action. They target and tame the inflammation in the airways, helping to prevent asthma symptoms and maintain long-term control. Popular examples include fluticasone, budesonide, and beclomethasone.

- **Long-Acting Beta-Agonists (LABA):**

  Long-acting beta-agonists work hand-in-hand with corticosteroids to provide sustained bronchodilation, keeping the airways relaxed for an extended period. Common LABAs include salmeterol and formoterol.

- **Leukotriene Modifiers:**

  Leukotriene modifiers, such as montelukast, zafirlukast, and zileuton, intervene in the inflammatory process by targeting leukotrienes. These are substances that play a role in triggering asthma symptoms.

- **Mast Cell Stabilizers:**

  Mast cell stabilizers, like cromolyn sodium, help prevent the release of substances that contribute to inflammation and bronchoconstriction. They are particularly useful in individuals with exercise-induced asthma.

Controllers are the cornerstone of asthma management, providing the foundation for long-term stability and control over asthma symptoms. By consistently taking controller medications as prescribed, individuals can significantly reduce the risk of asthma exacerbations and maintain optimal respiratory health.

What Are Relievers?

Relievers, as the name suggests, are the swift responders, stepping in to provide rapid relief when asthma symptoms rear their head. These medications are like the emergency responders of the respiratory world, quickly alleviating bronchoconstriction and making breathing easier. Relievers are typically short-acting bronchodilators, and they act by relaxing the muscles around the airways, opening them up for improved airflow.

Common types of reliever medications include:

- **Short-Acting Beta-Agonists (SABA):**

  Short-acting beta-agonists are the go-to medications for quick relief of acute asthma symptoms. Albuterol and levalbuterol are examples of SABAs. They act rapidly, providing relief within minutes.

- **Anticholinergics:**

  Short-acting anticholinergics, such as ipratropium bromide, work by blocking the action of acetylcholine, a neurotransmitter that can contribute to bronchoconstriction. These medications are often used in combination with SABAs for more comprehensive relief.

Relievers are crucial for managing acute symptoms, such as wheezing, shortness of breath, and chest tightness. However, it's important to note that relying on relievers alone without addressing underlying inflammation may lead to inadequate asthma control. For optimal management, relievers should be used as directed by healthcare providers and complemented by controller medications for long-term stability.

What Are Combination Medications?

Imagine a dynamic duo working in harmony to address both inflammation and bronchoconstriction – that's the power of combination medications. These formulations bring together the strengths of controllers and relievers in a single inhaler, simplifying the medication regimen for individuals with asthma. By combining the anti-inflammatory action of corticosteroids with the bronchodilation provided by long-acting beta-agonists, combination medications offer comprehensive asthma management.

Common types of combination medications include:

- **Inhaled Corticosteroid/Long-Acting Beta-Agonist (ICS/LABA):**

  This combination pairs the anti-inflammatory effects of inhaled corticosteroids with the sustained bronchodilation of long-acting beta-agonists. Examples include fluticasone/salmeterol and budesonide/formoterol.

- **Inhaled Corticosteroid/Long-Acting Muscarinic Antagonist (ICS/LAMA):**

  Some combination inhalers include long-acting muscarinic antagonists alongside corticosteroids. This combination addresses both inflammation and bronchoconstriction. Examples include fluticasone/umeclidinium/vilanterol.

Combination medications offer the convenience of a single inhaler while providing comprehensive asthma management. They are particularly beneficial for individuals who require both anti-inflammatory and bronchodilator medications to achieve optimal control.

What Effects Do Anti-Inflammatory Medications Have?

Anti-inflammatory medications are the peacekeepers, working diligently to soothe the inflammation in the airways and prevent the cascade of events that lead to asthma symptoms. Let's explore the effects of two key types of anti-inflammatory medications: inhaled corticosteroids and leukotriene modifiers.

- **Inhaled Corticosteroids (ICS):**

Inhaled corticosteroids are like the maestros orchestrating a symphony of anti-inflammatory effects in the airways. They work by:

  - **Reducing Inflammation:** ICS target and inhibit the inflammatory processes in the airways, preventing the release of substances that contribute to swelling and narrowing of the air passages.
  - **Decreasing Mucus Production:** By calming inflammation, ICS help reduce the production of thick mucus in the airways, making it easier to breathe.
  - **Preventing Airway Hyperresponsiveness:** ICS contribute to maintaining normal responsiveness of the airways, preventing excessive constriction in response to triggers.

Inhaled corticosteroids are a cornerstone of asthma management, offering sustained anti-inflammatory effects for long-term control.

- **Leukotriene Modifiers:**

Leukotriene modifiers take a different approach to anti-inflammatory action. They target leukotrienes, substances that play a role in triggering asthma symptoms. Leukotriene modifiers:

  - **Block Leukotriene Action:** By interfering with the action of leukotrienes, these medications help reduce inflammation and bronchoconstriction in the airways.
  - **Address Allergic Reactions:** Some leukotriene modifiers, such as montelukast, are particularly effective in managing asthma triggered by allergic reactions.
  - **Provide Long-Term Control:** Leukotriene modifiers are often used as part of a comprehensive asthma management plan, offering additional anti-inflammatory benefits.

Anti-inflammatory medications play a pivotal role in maintaining long-term asthma control. By addressing inflammation at its source, these medications contribute to reduced symptoms, improved lung function, and enhanced overall respiratory well-being.

What Effects Do Airway Opener Medications Have?

Airway opener medications, also known as bronchodilators, are the breath of fresh air when it comes to managing asthma symptoms. These medications act swiftly to relax the muscles around the airways, allowing for improved airflow and easier breathing. Let's delve into the effects of two key types of airway openers: short-acting beta-agonists (SABA) and anticholinergics.

- **Short-Acting Beta-Agonists (SABA):**

  SABAs are like the rescue squad, rushing to the scene to provide rapid relief during asthma flare-ups. These medications:

  - **Relax Airway Muscles:** SABAs act on beta receptors in the airway muscles, triggering relaxation and widening of the air passages.
  - **Prompt Onset of Action:** SABAs have a rapid onset of action, making them the go-to choice for quick relief during acute asthma symptoms.
  - **Improve Breathing Capacity:** By quickly opening up the airways, SABAs enhance breathing capacity and alleviate symptoms such as wheezing and shortness of breath.

  SABAs are a critical component of asthma management, providing the immediate relief needed during asthma attacks or exacerbations.

- **Anticholinergics:**

  Anticholinergics, such as ipratropium bromide, work by blocking the action of acetylcholine, a neurotransmitter that can contribute to bronchoconstriction. These medications:

  - **Induce Bronchodilation:** By inhibiting the effects of acetylcholine, anticholinergics induce bronchodilation, relaxing the muscles around the airways.
  - **Provide Additional Relief:** Anticholinergics may be used in combination with SABAs to provide additional relief during acute asthma symptoms.

- **Suitable for Some Individuals:** Anticholinergics are particularly beneficial for individuals who may not tolerate or adequately respond to SABAs alone.

Anticholinergics contribute to the bronchodilation needed for effective asthma symptom relief, complementing the action of SABAs.

What Are Glucocorticosteroids?

Enter the realm of glucocorticosteroids, often simply referred to as corticosteroids, and discover the potent anti-inflammatory power within. These medications, whether inhaled, oral, or intravenous form, harness the body's own anti-inflammatory processes to quell inflammation and restore balance to the airways.

Let's uncover the key aspects of glucocorticosteroids and their role in asthma management:

- **Inhaled Corticosteroids (ICS):**

  Inhaled corticosteroids are the frontline defenders against airway inflammation. These medications:

  - **Local Anti-Inflammatory Action:** ICS are delivered directly to the airways through inhalation, allowing for targeted anti-inflammatory action where it's needed most.
  - **Minimal Systemic Absorption:** The use of inhaled corticosteroids minimizes systemic absorption, reducing the risk of systemic side effects often associated with oral corticosteroids.
  - **Preventive and Long-Term Control:** ICS are a mainstay in preventive asthma care, providing long-term control and reducing the risk of exacerbations.
- **Oral and Intravenous Corticosteroids:**

  In certain situations, oral or intravenous corticosteroids may be prescribed for short-term use during severe asthma exacerbations. These medications:

  - **Potent Anti-Inflammatory Effects:** Oral and intravenous corticosteroids offer potent anti-inflammatory effects throughout the body, rapidly addressing widespread inflammation.

- **Reserved for Severe Exacerbations:** Due to the risk of systemic side effects, these forms of corticosteroids are typically reserved for short-term use during severe exacerbations that do not respond to other treatments.
- **Transition to Maintenance Therapy:** After a severe exacerbation, individuals may transition back to inhaled corticosteroids or other maintenance therapies for long-term asthma control.

Glucocorticosteroids, when used as part of a comprehensive asthma management plan, contribute to effective inflammation control, symptom relief, and improved overall respiratory health.

In conclusion, navigating the landscape of asthma medications involves understanding the roles of controllers, relievers, combination medications, anti-inflammatory wonders, airway openers, and the powerful realm of glucocorticosteroids. By embracing the diverse arsenal of medications available, individuals with asthma can tailor their treatment plans to achieve optimal control, leading to a life filled with breaths of ease and vitality. Always consult with healthcare providers to determine the most suitable medications for your individual needs and ensure a personalized approach to asthma management.

The Symphony of Breath: Understanding Asthma Medications Beyond the Mist

Welcome to the symphony of breath, where the spotlight shines on glucocorticosteroids, tablets that play a different tune, the intriguing dance of corticosteroids and anabolic steroids, the melody of inhaled non-steroidal anti-inflammatory medications, the quest for alternatives to inhaled corticosteroids, and the lingering question of whether you still need your inhaler when you feel okay. In this chapter, we unravel the mysteries behind these medications, demystifying their roles in the grand performance of asthma management.

Why Are Glucocorticosteroid Medications Inhaled?

Enter the stage of inhaled glucocorticosteroids, the superheroes of localized anti-inflammatory action. But why the inhalation route? Let's pull back the curtain on this theatrical choice.

- **Targeted Action:**

  Inhaled glucocorticosteroids are like precision artists, delivering their anti-inflammatory magic directly to the airways where it's needed most. This targeted action minimizes systemic absorption, reducing the risk of side effects compared to oral or injectable forms.

- **Airway Defense:**

  The inhaled route allows these medications to establish a defense line right where inflammation brews – in the airways. By taming the inflammatory response at its source, inhaled glucocorticosteroids contribute to long-term asthma control.

- **Minimized Side Effects:**

  Inhaled administration minimizes the exposure of other body tissues to corticosteroids, focusing their effects on the respiratory system. This helps avoid the broad systemic side effects associated with oral or injectable corticosteroids.

- **Patient Convenience:**

  Inhalation is a convenient and patient-friendly method. It allows individuals to self-administer their medication, enhancing adherence to treatment plans and promoting a sense of empowerment in asthma management.

Inhaled glucocorticosteroids, with their targeted and localized action, take center stage in preventing and managing airway inflammation, offering a breath of relief without the full orchestra of systemic effects.

When and Why Are Corticosteroid Tablets or Injections Used?

While inhaled glucocorticosteroids often steal the spotlight, there are moments when corticosteroid tablets or injections take a dramatic turn in the asthma management narrative.

- **Severe Exacerbations:**

  Corticosteroid tablets or injections come into play during severe asthma exacerbations, when the need for rapid and widespread anti-inflammatory action is paramount. In these critical moments, oral or injectable corticosteroids offer a potent response to quell inflammation throughout the body.

- **Limited Duration:**

  The use of corticosteroid tablets or injections is typically of short duration, addressing acute exacerbations and providing swift relief. Prolonged use of systemic corticosteroids comes with an increased risk of side effects, making them unsuitable for long-term asthma control.

- **Transition from Acute to Maintenance Therapy:**

  After the storm of a severe exacerbation subsides, individuals may transition back to inhaled glucocorticosteroids or other maintenance therapies for long-term asthma control. Systemic corticosteroids serve as a bridge during these challenging moments.

- **Individualized Approach:**

  The decision to use corticosteroid tablets or injections is made based on the severity of the exacerbation and individual health considerations. Healthcare providers carefully weigh the benefits and risks to tailor treatment plans to each patient's unique needs.

While systemic corticosteroids offer powerful anti-inflammatory effects during critical episodes, their use is circumscribed to specific situations, and their prolonged deployment is approached with caution due to potential side effects.

What Is the Difference Between a Corticosteroid and an Anabolic Steroid?

The theater of steroids unfolds, revealing two distinct characters – corticosteroids and anabolic steroids. Let's illuminate the stage with the key differences between these players in the steroid saga.

- **Corticosteroids:**
    - **Nature's Architects:** Corticosteroids, including glucocorticosteroids used in asthma management, are naturally occurring hormones produced by the adrenal glands.
    - **Anti-Inflammatory Maestros:** Corticosteroids play a crucial role in regulating inflammation, immune responses, and metabolic processes in the body.
    - **Asthma Allies:** In the context of asthma, corticosteroids act as anti-inflammatory agents, reducing airway inflammation and preventing asthma symptoms.
- **Anabolic Steroids:**
    - **Synthetic Compounds:** Anabolic steroids are synthetic variations of the male sex hormone testosterone.
    - **Muscle Builders:** Anabolic steroids are often associated with muscle-building effects and are used illicitly in some cases to enhance athletic performance.
    - **Not Asthma Medications:** Unlike corticosteroids used in asthma management, anabolic steroids are not prescribed for the treatment of asthma. Their use outside medical supervision can lead to serious health risks.

While both corticosteroids and anabolic steroids fall under the umbrella of steroids, their roles, origins, and applications are distinctly different. Corticosteroids are the protagonists in the asthma narrative, offering anti-inflammatory prowess for respiratory wellness.

What Are Inhaled Non-Steroidal Anti-Inflammatory Medications?

In the world of asthma management, the spotlight isn't solely reserved for steroids. Inhaled non-steroidal anti-inflammatory medications step into the limelight, offering an alternative route to address airway inflammation without the corticosteroid touch.

- **Leukotriene Modifiers:**
  - **Targeting Leukotrienes:** Inhaled non-steroidal anti-inflammatory medications, particularly leukotriene modifiers like montelukast, intervene in the inflammatory process by targeting leukotrienes.
  - **Reducing Inflammation:** By blocking the action of leukotrienes, these medications help reduce inflammation and bronchoconstriction in the airways.
- **Mast Cell Stabilizers:**
  - **Preventing Release of Substances:** Mast cell stabilizers, such as cromolyn sodium, work by preventing the release of substances that contribute to inflammation and bronchoconstriction.
  - **Exercise-Induced Asthma:** These medications are particularly useful in individuals with exercise-induced asthma, providing preventive benefits.

Inhaled non-steroidal anti-inflammatory medications offer an alternative approach to asthma management, providing options for individuals who may have specific considerations or preferences regarding corticosteroid use.

Is There an Effective Alternative to Using Inhaled Corticosteroids?

The quest for alternatives to inhaled corticosteroids leads us to explore additional avenues in the asthma management landscape. While inhaled corticosteroids are cornerstone medications, some individuals may seek alternatives or complementary strategies.

- **Leukotriene Modifiers:**
  - **Alternative or Add-On Therapy:** Leukotriene modifiers, available in oral form, can serve as an alternative or add-on therapy for individuals who prefer options beyond inhaled corticosteroids.
- **Biologics:**
  - **Targeting Specific Pathways:** Biologic medications, such as monoclonal antibodies, target specific pathways involved in the inflammatory process. These medications are typically reserved for individuals with severe asthma unresponsive to traditional therapies.
- **Allergen Immunotherapy:**
  - **Addressing Allergies at the Source:** Allergen immunotherapy involves exposing individuals to small, controlled amounts of allergens to desensitize the immune system. This approach may be beneficial for individuals with asthma triggered by specific allergens.
- **Bronchial Thermoplasty:**
  - **Modulating Airway Smooth Muscle:** Bronchial thermoplasty is a procedure that applies controlled heat to the airway walls, reducing the smooth muscle mass and decreasing airway responsiveness. It is considered for individuals with severe asthma.

While inhaled corticosteroids remain the gold standard for asthma control, alternative and complementary options exist. The decision to explore alternatives should be made in consultation with healthcare providers, considering individual health needs and treatment goals.

Do I Still Need My Inhaled Corticosteroid If I Feel OK?
The finale of this chapter addresses a common question – whether to continue inhaled corticosteroids when asthma symptoms are at bay. Let's unravel the rationale behind this consideration.

- **Preventive Nature:**
  - **Maintaining Control:** Inhaled corticosteroids are preventive medications designed to maintain long-term control and prevent asthma symptoms, exacerbations, and airway inflammation.
  - **Consistency is Key:** Even when feeling well, continuing inhaled corticosteroids as prescribed helps sustain the baseline control necessary for respiratory wellness.

- **Risk of Relapse:**
  - **Underlying Inflammation:** Asthma involves chronic airway inflammation, even when symptoms are not actively manifesting. Discontinuing inhaled corticosteroids may lead to a resurgence of inflammation, making it challenging to regain control quickly if symptoms reappear.
- **Individualized Approach:**
  - **Consultation with Healthcare Providers:** Decisions regarding the continuation or adjustment of inhaled corticosteroids should be made in consultation with healthcare providers. They can assess individual health status, monitor lung function, and tailor treatment plans based on the specific needs of each patient.

In summary, the role of inhaled corticosteroids extends beyond symptom relief; it encompasses the maintenance of long-term control and prevention of future exacerbations. By embracing these medications as a consistent part of asthma management, individuals can breathe with confidence, knowing they are proactively safeguarding their respiratory health.

As the curtain falls on this chapter, the tapestry of asthma medications unfolds with clarity. From inhaled glucocorticosteroids to systemic corticosteroids, non-steroidal anti-inflammatory medications, and the quest for alternatives, each element plays a vital role in the symphony of asthma management. Through understanding and collaboration with healthcare providers, individuals can navigate the complexities of medication choices, ensuring a harmonious and empowering journey towards optimal respiratory well-being.

A Breath of Relief: Addressing Asthma and Beyond

In the symphony of health, asthma can sometimes be accompanied by other challenges like strained muscles, aching joints, severe back pain, or rheumatism. This chapter aims to be your guide through the labyrinth of anti-inflammatory solutions for these common woes, introducing the concept of hyposensitization, and providing practical tips for when asthma acts up in the chilly embrace of cold weather.

Anti-Inflammatory Medications in Asthma: A Balancing Act

When asthma shares the stage with strained muscles, aching joints, or other inflammatory conditions, finding the right anti-inflammatory medication becomes crucial. While certain medications may exacerbate asthma symptoms, there are alternatives that can offer relief without compromising respiratory health.

- **Acetaminophen (Paracetamol):**
  - *Pain Management Ally:* Acetaminophen is a go-to option for pain management and fever reduction.
  - *Asthma-Friendly:* It is generally considered safe for individuals with asthma as it lacks the anti-inflammatory properties that some other medications possess.
- **NSAIDs (Nonsteroidal Anti-Inflammatory Drugs):**
  - *Proceed with Caution:* While NSAIDs like ibuprofen are effective for pain relief, they can worsen asthma symptoms in some individuals.
  - *Individual Response Varies:* It's essential to be vigilant and monitor how your body responds to NSAIDs. If they trigger asthma symptoms, consult your healthcare provider for alternatives.
- **Topical Analgesics:**
  - *Localized Relief:* Creams, gels, or patches containing NSAIDs or other pain-relieving ingredients offer localized relief without the systemic effects that oral medications can have.
  - *Consideration for Asthma:* Topical analgesics may be a suitable option for individuals cautious about the potential impact of oral medications on asthma.

- **Corticosteroid Injections:**
    - *Targeted Relief:* In cases of severe pain or inflammation, corticosteroid injections can provide targeted relief to specific areas.
    - *Short-Term Use:* These injections are typically used for short-term relief due to the potential for side effects with prolonged use.

Choosing the right anti-inflammatory approach involves a nuanced understanding of individual health considerations, including asthma status. Consult with your healthcare provider to tailor a solution that addresses both your pain and asthma management needs.

Hyposensitization (Vaccination): Nurturing Immune Harmony

Hyposensitization, often likened to vaccination, is a unique approach that aims to recalibrate the immune system's response to allergens. Let's unravel this concept and explore how it can bring relief to individuals troubled by allergies, including allergic asthma.

- **Understanding Allergic Sensitivities:**
    - *Immune Overreaction:* Allergies, including allergic asthma, occur when the immune system overreacts to harmless substances, triggering symptoms like wheezing, sneezing, or itching.
- **Essence of Hyposensitization:**
    - *Building Tolerance:* Hyposensitization involves exposing individuals to small, controlled amounts of allergens to desensitize the immune system gradually.
    - *Allergen Desensitization:* Over time, the immune system becomes less responsive to these allergens, reducing the intensity of allergic reactions.
- **Forms of Hyposensitization:**
    - *Subcutaneous Immunotherapy (SCIT):* Allergen extracts are injected under the skin, usually by healthcare providers.
    - *Sublingual Immunotherapy (SLIT):* Allergen extracts are placed under the tongue in the form of drops or tablets, often self-administered.
- **Conditions Addressed by Hyposensitization:**
    - *Allergic Rhinitis (Hay Fever):* Common allergens like pollen, dust mites, and pet dander.
    - *Allergic Asthma:* Asthma triggered by specific allergens.

Hyposensitization offers a promising pathway to long-term relief for individuals burdened by allergic reactions. It requires commitment, but the potential benefits can significantly improve quality of life.

Tackling Cold Weather Woes: Asthma Outdoors

Cold weather can pose challenges for individuals with asthma, but with some thoughtful strategies, you can navigate the outdoors with greater ease.

- **Bundle Up:**
  - *Wardrobe Arsenal:* Dress warmly to protect yourself from the cold. Layering is key, and don't forget hats and gloves to retain body heat.
- **Use a Scarf or Mask:**
  - *Warm Air Shield:* Cover your nose and mouth with a scarf or mask to help humidify and warm the air before it enters your airways.
- **Preventive Medication Use:**
  - *Stay Consistent:* Ensure you use your preventive asthma medications as prescribed, especially before heading outdoors in cold weather.
- **Stay Active Indoors:**
  - *Indoor Alternatives:* Engage in indoor physical activities to maintain overall health and fitness during colder months.
- **Monitor Symptoms:**
  - *Be Attentive:* Pay attention to any signs of shortness of breath, wheezing, or chest tightness when exposed to cold air.
  - *Prompt Action:* If symptoms occur, take prompt action by using reliever medications as prescribed.

By incorporating these simple yet effective strategies, individuals with asthma can not only survive but thrive in the crisp embrace of cold weather.

In closing, this chapter is a compass to navigate the diverse landscapes of health, providing practical insights for addressing pain and inflammation, demystifying hyposensitization, and offering solutions for enjoying the great outdoors even in chilly weather. May this knowledge empower you to breathe freely and live vibrantly.

Chapter 7

Asthma: Side Effects, Medications, and Long-Term Well-being

Answers following Questions:
Can asthma itself cause side effects?
Can tiredness and forgetfulness be caused by my asthma medication?
Do inhaled corticosteroids cause any long-term side effects?
Is it good for me to always use inhaled corticosteroids?
Can I become addicted to the corticosteroids in asthma medications?
Why can I use inhaled corticosteroids for many years, but corticosteroid cream on my skin for only a short period?
Do I need to rinse out my mouth after using an inhaled corticosteroid?
If I can't remember whether I actually took my daily maintenance dose of inhaled corticosteroid, is it better to risk taking a double dose or none at all?
What can I do to prevent osteoporosis?

Side Effects, Medications, and Long-Term Well-being

In the intricate tapestry of asthma management, understanding the nuances of side effects, medication concerns, and long-term well-being is paramount. This chapter aims to demystify common questions regarding side effects from asthma itself, the impact of medications on tiredness and forgetfulness, the long-term implications of inhaled corticosteroids, and essential considerations for maintaining overall health. Let's embark on this journey to empower individuals with asthma and their caregivers.

Can Asthma Itself Cause Side Effects?

Asthma, in its essence, is a chronic condition that affects the airways, and while the primary symptoms involve difficulty breathing, coughing, and wheezing, asthma itself doesn't typically cause side effects in the traditional sense. However, the challenges of living with asthma can bring about certain experiences that might be perceived as side effects:

- **Fatigue:** The effort required to breathe during asthma exacerbations can lead to fatigue.
- **Emotional Impact:** Living with a chronic condition may contribute to stress or anxiety, influencing emotional well-being.

Addressing these aspects is integral to holistic asthma management. Effective control measures, emotional support, and lifestyle adjustments can help minimize these perceived side effects.

Can Tiredness and Forgetfulness Be Caused by My Asthma Medication?

A common concern among individuals using asthma medications revolves around the potential side effects of tiredness and forgetfulness. It's crucial to recognize that various asthma medications may affect individuals differently, and the impact on energy levels and cognitive functions can vary:

- **Bronchodilators:** Short-acting bronchodilators, while essential for relieving acute symptoms, may cause temporary jitteriness or increased heart rate in some individuals.

- **Oral Corticosteroids:** Systemic corticosteroids, often prescribed for severe exacerbations, may lead to temporary side effects like mood changes or difficulty concentrating.

If you experience persistent tiredness or forgetfulness, it's essential to discuss these concerns with your healthcare provider. They can assess your medication regimen, explore alternative options, or provide guidance on managing potential side effects.

Do Inhaled Corticosteroids Cause Any Long-Term Side Effects?

Inhaled corticosteroids (ICS) are cornerstone medications for managing asthma, prized for their effectiveness in reducing airway inflammation. Concerns about long-term side effects are valid, but it's crucial to weigh the benefits against potential risks:

- **Bone Health:** Long-term use of high doses of ICS may slightly increase the risk of osteoporosis, affecting bone density.
- **Cataracts and Glaucoma:** Prolonged use, especially at high doses, may marginally elevate the risk of cataracts and glaucoma.

It's important to note that the benefits of controlling asthma and preventing exacerbations often outweigh the potential risks. Regular follow-ups with healthcare providers, bone density assessments, and open communication about concerns ensure a balanced approach to asthma management.

Is It Good for Me to Always Use Inhaled Corticosteroids?

Consistent use of inhaled corticosteroids is essential for maintaining long-term asthma control and preventing exacerbations. These medications:

- **Control Inflammation:** ICS target airway inflammation, reducing the frequency and severity of asthma symptoms.
- **Prevent Exacerbations:** Regular use minimizes the risk of acute exacerbations, leading to improved quality of life.
- **Maintain Lung Function:** ICS contribute to preserving lung function over time.

While concerns about long-term use exist, the benefits of stable asthma control typically outweigh potential risks. Healthcare providers tailor treatment plans based on individual needs, adjusting medication dosages as required.

Can I Become Addicted to the Corticosteroids in Asthma Medications?

The fear of addiction to corticosteroids is a common misconception. In the context of asthma medications, particularly inhaled corticosteroids, addiction doesn't apply. Corticosteroids used for asthma are not addictive, and discontinuing them doesn't lead to withdrawal symptoms associated with addiction.

Why Can I Use Inhaled Corticosteroids for Many Years, but Corticosteroid Cream on My Skin for Only a Short Period?

The distinction in duration of use between inhaled corticosteroids and corticosteroid creams lies in the nature of application and absorption:

- **Localized vs. Systemic:** Inhaled corticosteroids primarily target the airways, leading to minimal systemic absorption and side effects. On the contrary, corticosteroid creams applied to the skin have higher absorption rates, potentially causing systemic effects over prolonged use.
- **Risk-Benefit Ratio:** The decision to limit the duration of corticosteroid cream use is often based on the risk-benefit ratio, balancing the therapeutic benefits with the potential for side effects.

It's crucial to follow healthcare provider recommendations regarding the duration and application of corticosteroid creams, ensuring optimal therapeutic outcomes while minimizing potential risks.

Do I Need to Rinse Out My Mouth After Using an Inhaled Corticosteroid?

Rinsing the mouth after using an inhaled corticosteroid is a recommended practice for several reasons:

- **Oral Candidiasis Prevention:** Inhaled corticosteroids may contribute to the overgrowth of Candida (yeast) in the mouth, leading to oral candidiasis or thrush.

- **Minimizing Local Side Effects:** Rinsing helps remove residual medication from the mouth, reducing the risk of local side effects such as hoarseness or throat irritation.

Simple practices like rinsing with water or using a mouthwash after inhaler use can significantly mitigate these potential side effects.

If I Can't Remember Whether I Actually Took My Daily Maintenance Dose of Inhaled Corticosteroid, Is It Better to Risk Taking a Double Dose or None at All?

The dilemma of whether to take a double dose or skip a dose when faced with uncertainty is a common concern. The recommended approach varies based on individual circumstances:

- **Missing a Dose:**
  - If unsure, it's generally safer to skip the dose if taking a double dose poses potential risks.
  - Missing an occasional dose is unlikely to significantly impact asthma control.
- **Consulting Healthcare Providers:**
  - If uncertain about the appropriate course of action, seek guidance from your healthcare provider.
  - They can provide personalized recommendations based on your asthma management plan.

Consistency is key in asthma management, but occasional missed doses can be addressed without compromising overall control. Open communication with healthcare providers ensures a tailored approach to such situations.

What Can I Do to Prevent Osteoporosis?

Osteoporosis, characterized by decreased bone density and an increased risk of fractures, is a concern for individuals using long-term corticosteroids, especially at high doses. Practical strategies to prevent osteoporosis include:

- **Adequate Calcium Intake:** Ensure a diet rich in calcium through dairy products, leafy greens, and fortified foods.
- **Vitamin D Supplementation:** Maintain optimal vitamin D levels through sunlight exposure and, if necessary, supplements.

- **Regular Weight-Bearing Exercise:** Engage in weight-bearing exercises like walking or strength training to support bone health.
- **Bone Density Monitoring:** Periodic bone density assessments help identify changes early, allowing for proactive interventions.

These measures, combined with open communication with healthcare providers, contribute to comprehensive osteoporosis prevention for individuals using corticosteroids.

Chapter 8
Asthma & Infections

Answers following Questions:
Do infections cause asthma?
Do infections trigger asthma?
Why don't antibiotics help against asthmatic inflammation in the airways?
Is asthma contagious?

Do Infections Cause Asthma? Unraveling the Connection

In the journey through the intricate maze of asthma, one often wonders about the role infections play in this respiratory condition. Does catching a cold pave the way for asthma, and if so, why? Why do antibiotics seem powerless against the wheezing and breathlessness that asthma brings? Is asthma something you can catch from someone like the common cold? Let's embark on a journey through the web of infections and asthma, demystifying the connection in a language that speaks to all.

Infections and Asthma: A Dance of Triggers

Do Infections Trigger Asthma?

Imagine your body as a bustling city, with its defense system always on high alert. Now, picture an infection marching into this city, armed with its own set of challenges. This clash between the body's defense and the invading infection can be a trigger for asthma, especially in those who are already prone to the condition.

Infections like the common cold or the flu can sometimes set off a chain reaction, leading to inflammation in the airways. For some individuals, this inflammation might just be a passing inconvenience, but for those with asthma, it can be the spark that ignites the wheezing and tightness in the chest.

Why Don't Antibiotics Help Against Asthmatic Inflammation?

Ah, antibiotics – the superheroes of the medical world. But wait, why don't they swoop in to save the day when it comes to asthma triggered by infections?

Picture this: antibiotics are like skilled carpenters equipped to fix a leaky roof. They are experts at tackling bacterial infections, but asthma triggered by infections often involves a different culprit – viruses. Antibiotics, unfortunately, are powerless against these viral invaders. So, when it's a viral infection provoking your asthma symptoms, antibiotics might as well be trying to fix a leaky roof with a paintbrush.

Understanding the enemy is crucial, and in the case of asthma triggered by infections, knowing whether it's a bacterium or a virus calling the shots helps in choosing the right weapon.

Dispelling Myths: Is Asthma Contagious?

Is Asthma Contagious?

Let's put it bluntly — no, asthma is not contagious. You can't catch it like you catch a cold from a friend's sneeze or a doorknob that has been touched by too many hands.

Asthma is more like a unique fingerprint, individualized and shaped by a combination of genetic and environmental factors. While infections can sometimes act as triggers for asthma symptoms, asthma itself doesn't spread from person to person through a casual encounter.

So, if your friend has asthma, you can still share a hug without fear. Asthma isn't looking for new hosts; it's a condition that develops in individuals based on their own distinct set of circumstances.

A Closing Note: Navigating the Intersection of Infections and Asthma

As we wrap up this chapter, it's crucial to remember that the relationship between infections and asthma is like a complex dance. Sometimes infections can step on asthma's toes, leading to a symphony of wheezing and coughing. Other times, your body's defense might gracefully navigate through an infection without triggering an asthma episode.

Understanding this dance empowers individuals and their caregivers to take proactive steps. Recognizing the signs, seeking timely medical advice, and being aware of the limitations of antibiotics can all contribute to a smoother choreography in the intricate ballet of infections and asthma.

Chapter 9

Breathing Easy While Breaking a Sweat: Navigating Exercise with Asthma

Answers following Questions:

Is it good for people with asthma to exercise?

Exercise is good for you. So why can it cause asthma symptoms?

How can I avoid exercise-induced asthma?

Are some kinds of physical activities more suitable for people with asthma?

How intensively do I dare to exercise?

I often feel my asthma when I jog. Do I have to quit jogging?

What should I do if I get asthma symptoms while exercising?

Can I take asthma medications and still take part in competitive sports?

In the grand tapestry of health, few threads are as brightly colored as regular exercise. We often hear about the myriad benefits: improved heart health, better mood, and even a boost in overall well-being. But what about those who bear the tag of asthma? Can they partake in this healthful endeavor without fear? Let's explore the relationship between exercise and asthma in a language that speaks directly to you, the reader.

Embracing the Benefits: Why Exercise Matters

Exercise is Good for You. So Why Can it Cause Asthma Symptoms?

First things first, let's establish a simple truth: exercise is good for everyone, including those with asthma. It gets the heart pumping, the muscles working, and the entire body humming along like a well-tuned engine.

Now, here's the catch. Sometimes, for individuals with asthma, exercise can act like a mischievous imp, triggering symptoms such as coughing, wheezing, and shortness of breath. It's not the exercise itself that's the culprit, but how the body reacts to the increased activity. Think of it as your body's way of saying, "Hey, I need a bit more support here!"

Why Does Exercise Trigger Asthma Symptoms?

To unravel this mystery, let's delve into the intricate workings of the respiratory system. When you exercise, your breathing rate increases, and you take in more air. For some individuals with asthma, this heightened activity can lead to the release of substances that cause inflammation in the airways.

Additionally, the airways may become more sensitive, reacting to triggers that wouldn't normally provoke a response. This heightened sensitivity can contribute to the symptoms experienced during or after exercise.

Navigating the Path: Tips for Exercising with Asthma

How Can I Avoid Exercise-Induced Asthma?

The good news is, there's no need to bid farewell to your favorite physical activities. Instead, let's lace up those sneakers and explore ways to avoid the unwelcome guest known as exercise-induced asthma.

- **Warm-Up Wisely:** Before diving headfirst into your exercise routine, warm up gradually. This prepares your body for the increased activity and may help stave off asthma symptoms.
- **Choose Your Battle:** Opt for activities that are less likely to trigger asthma. Swimming, walking, or cycling are often gentler on the respiratory system than high-intensity sports.
- **Breathe Right:** Pay attention to your breathing technique. Slow, controlled breaths can help prevent rapid breathing, a common trigger for asthma during exercise.
- **Know Your Limits:** While pushing your boundaries is encouraged, it's crucial to know your limits. Pushing too hard, too fast can increase the risk of asthma symptoms.

Tailoring the Routine: Asthma-Friendly Physical Activities

Are Some Kinds of Physical Activities More Suitable for People with Asthma?

Absolutely. Consider this your invitation to a world of exercise where asthma can peacefully coexist. Activities that involve steady, rhythmic movements tend to be more asthma-friendly. Swimming, yoga, and brisk walking are excellent choices, allowing you to reap the rewards of exercise without provoking your asthma.

The Aquatic Symphony: Swimming as an Asthma-Friendly Exercise

Dive into the calm waters of swimming, and you'll find a haven for your lungs. The humid environment can be gentler on the respiratory system, and the rhythmic strokes provide a cardiovascular workout without the high impact.

Yoga: A Breath of Serenity

Enter the world of yoga, where each pose is a dance of breath and movement. Yoga not only enhances flexibility and strength but also encourages mindful breathing. This can be particularly beneficial for individuals with asthma, promoting a sense of calm and control.

The Joy of Walking: A Simple and Effective Exercise

For those seeking a straightforward yet powerful exercise, walking is a timeless choice. It's low impact, easily customizable, and allows you to enjoy the great outdoors while giving your cardiovascular system a gentle workout.

Setting the Pace: How Intensively Do I Dare to Exercise?

How Intensively Do I Dare to Exercise?

The golden rule here is to listen to your body. Push yourself, but not to the point of exhaustion. Aim for a pace that allows you to hold a conversation without gasping for breath. Gradually building up intensity over time can also help your body adjust, reducing the likelihood of asthma symptoms.

High-Intensity vs. Low-Intensity Exercise: Finding Your Sweet Spot

While high-intensity exercise can indeed trigger asthma symptoms, it doesn't mean you're confined to a realm of low-intensity activities. It's about finding the balance that works for you. Some individuals with asthma can comfortably engage in high-intensity workouts with proper management and gradual progression.

Jogging Dilemmas: I Often Feel My Asthma When I Jog. Do I Have to Quit Jogging?

Do I Have to Quit Jogging?

Fear not, jogging enthusiasts. While jogging can sometimes trigger asthma symptoms, it doesn't mean you have to hang up your running shoes for good. Consider adjusting your pace, incorporating walking intervals, or exploring other forms of cardiovascular exercise. Finding the right balance allows you to enjoy the benefits of jogging without the unwelcome wheezing.

Tips for Jogging with Asthma: A Breath-by-Breath Guide

- **Warm Up with a Walk:** Begin your jogging session with a brisk walk to gradually elevate your heart rate.
- **Incorporate Intervals:** Mix jogging with walking intervals to reduce the overall intensity and give your respiratory system a chance to adapt.
- **Choose Optimal Conditions:** Pick times and locations with favorable air quality and moderate temperatures to minimize potential triggers.
- **Stay Hydrated:** Proper hydration helps maintain the elasticity of airways, potentially reducing the risk of asthma symptoms.

On the Spot Solutions: Dealing with Asthma Symptoms During Exercise

What Should I Do if I Get Asthma Symptoms While Exercising?
Imagine you're midway through your workout, and here comes that familiar wheeze. What now? First and foremost, don't panic. Find a quiet spot, take slow and steady breaths, and if you have a rescue inhaler, use it as directed. If symptoms persist, it's essential to seek medical advice. Your healthcare team can provide personalized guidance to ensure your exercise routine aligns with your asthma management plan.

Creating an Emergency Action Plan: Your Asthma Toolkit

- **Rescue Inhaler:** Always carry your rescue inhaler, and ensure it's easily accessible during exercise.
- **Identify Triggers:** Be aware of environmental factors that may trigger your asthma and try to avoid them during exercise.
- **Emergency Contact:** Share your exercise plans with someone close, so they're aware and can assist in case of an emergency.
- **Know When to Stop:** If symptoms worsen or persist, it's crucial to stop exercising and seek medical attention promptly.

Competing with Confidence: Asthma Medications and Competitive Sports

Can I Take Asthma Medications and Still Take Part in Competitive Sports?
Absolutely. Asthma should never be a barrier to pursuing your athletic dreams. Many successful athletes manage asthma while competing at the highest levels. The key is effective asthma management, including adherence to prescribed medications and open communication with your healthcare team. With the right support, you can conquer both the track and the challenges asthma may present.

Balancing Act: Medications and Athletic Performance
Understanding how asthma medications work is key to striking the right balance between managing your symptoms and excelling in your chosen sport.

- **Bronchodilators:** These medications help open up the airways, making it easier to breathe. They are often used before exercise to prevent symptoms.

- **Anti-Inflammatory Medications:** Long-term control medications help reduce inflammation in the airways, providing a foundation for stable asthma management.
- **Personalized Approach:** Work closely with your healthcare team to tailor your medication plan to your specific needs and the demands of your chosen sport.

In concluding this extensive exploration, remember this: asthma doesn't have to bench you from the game of life. Embrace the benefits of exercise, listen to your body, and work hand-in-hand with your healthcare team to tailor a fitness routine that suits you. Whether you prefer the rhythmic strokes of swimming or the gentle cadence of a walk, the path to a healthier, more active life with asthma is yours to navigate.

Chapter 10

Exploring the Intersections of Asthma with Other Conditions

Answers following Questions:
Is asthma related to other chronic diseases, such as rheumatism and diabetes?
Is asthma a psychological (psychosomatic) disease?
What is the difference between asthma and COPD (chronic obstructive lung disease)?
Is emphysema the same as asthma?

Exploring the Intersections of Asthma with Other Conditions

In the vast landscape of health, it's natural to wonder about the connections between asthma and other chronic companions. Does asthma hold hands with conditions like rheumatism or diabetes? Is it more than just a physical challenge, stretching into the realm of the mind? And what about its distant cousin, COPD? Join me as we navigate these questions, shedding light on the intricate relationships that asthma has with other health players.

Connections Beyond Breath: Asthma and Other Chronic Diseases

Is Asthma Related to Other Chronic Diseases, Such as Rheumatism and Diabetes?

Let's embark on a journey through the intricate web of health. Asthma, while primarily a respiratory condition, can sometimes be found in the company of other chronic conditions like rheumatism (arthritis) or diabetes.

The Rheumatism Connection: Rheumatism, with its joint-related challenges, might seem like an unlikely partner for asthma. However, emerging research suggests that inflammation, a common thread in both conditions, could be the link. Understanding this connection allows healthcare teams to tailor treatment plans that address the complexities of coexisting conditions.

The Dance with Diabetes: On the other side of the spectrum, diabetes and asthma share the stage in unexpected ways. Both conditions involve inflammation, and certain medications used to manage diabetes may impact asthma symptoms. It's like a delicate dance where the rhythm of one condition influences the steps of the other.

In essence, while asthma has its own spotlight, it sometimes engages in a dance with other chronic conditions. This emphasizes the importance of a holistic approach to healthcare, where the interconnectedness of various conditions is considered in crafting a personalized treatment plan.

Mind and Breath: Is Asthma a Psychological (Psychosomatic) Disease?

Is Asthma a Psychological (Psychosomatic) Disease?

The mind-body connection is a fascinating realm, and when it comes to asthma, the question often arises: Is it more than just a physical ailment? While asthma is rooted in the respiratory system, the influence of the mind on its symptoms is not to be underestimated.

The Role of Stress: Imagine stress as an orchestra conductor, waving its baton and influencing the tempo of your body's responses. In the case of asthma, stress can be a powerful maestro, potentially triggering or exacerbating symptoms. It's not that asthma is solely in the mind, but rather, the mind can influence the symphony of symptoms.

The Emotional Breath: Emotions, like characters in a play, can also take center stage. Strong emotions, be they excitement or anxiety, can sometimes provoke asthma symptoms. Understanding this emotional interplay empowers individuals and their caregivers to navigate the emotional landscape while managing asthma effectively.

So, while asthma has its roots in the respiratory system, its branches can sway in the winds of emotions and stress. A holistic approach to asthma care acknowledges the influence of the mind, ensuring a well-rounded strategy for managing both the physical and emotional aspects.

What is the Difference Between Asthma and COPD (Chronic Obstructive Lung Disease)?

In the respiratory arena, two players often share the spotlight: asthma and chronic obstructive pulmonary disease (COPD). While they may appear similar, they have distinct characteristics that set them apart.

Asthma: The Flexible Performer: Asthma is like a flexible gymnast, capable of reversible airflow obstruction. This means that the constriction of airways that occurs during an asthma attack is, to a large extent, reversible with proper treatment. It often begins in childhood and can manifest as recurrent episodes of wheezing, coughing, and breathlessness.

COPD: The Irreversible Settler: On the other hand, COPD is more like a seasoned traveler, leaving irreversible damage in its wake. Typically, COPD develops later in life, often due to prolonged exposure to irritating gases or particulate matter (such as from smoking). The damage to the airways and lungs is progressive and tends to worsen over time.

Understanding these distinctions is crucial, as it guides healthcare professionals in tailoring treatment plans. While asthma responds well to medications that open the airways, COPD management involves a focus on slowing down the progression of irreversible damage.

Is Emphysema the Same as Asthma?

In the respiratory lexicon, terms like emphysema and asthma may sound like distant cousins, but they inhabit different realms of the respiratory landscape.

Emphysema: The Lung Architect's Dilemma: Emphysema is like a wayward architect, impacting the structural integrity of the lungs. In this condition, the air sacs (alveoli) lose their elasticity, making it challenging for the lungs to exhale air effectively. It's a common companion to COPD and often results from long-term exposure to harmful substances, most notably cigarette smoke.

Asthma: The Airway's Ebb and Flow: Asthma, in contrast, is more like a dynamic river. It involves reversible airway obstruction, where the smooth muscles surrounding the airways tighten (bronchoconstriction), leading to symptoms like wheezing and shortness of breath. Unlike emphysema, the airways in asthma can return to their normal state with the right treatment.

So, while emphysema and asthma may share the respiratory stage, they play different roles. Emphysema is a structural challenge, affecting the architecture of the lungs, while asthma is a reversible ebb and flow of airway dynamics.

As we wrap up this chapter, remember that the journey through health is a nuanced one. Asthma, with its intricate connections to other chronic conditions, beckons us to approach its management with a broad perspective. It's not merely a matter of addressing the physical symptoms but understanding the emotional and interconnected aspects as well.

Chapter 11
Navigating Life with Asthma

Answers following Questions:
What climate is best for a person with asthma?
Are relaxing exercises good for my asthma?
Is there a good breathing technique to use when my asthma symptoms get worse?
How does asthma affect my choice of a professional career?
Sometimes people have trouble understanding that I can't cope with perfumes and smoke. What can I do?
What can I do to improve my home environment in general?
Can I have pets even though I have asthma?
When I went to Spain on holiday I felt great – should I move there?
My asthma means that I have to miss out on activities that are important to me, such as dancing. This makes me sad and angry. What can I do?

Navigating Life with Asthma

In the kaleidoscope of life with asthma, questions often arise about the ideal climate, the role of exercise, and the impact on career choices. Additionally, the challenge of making others understand the unique struggles, such as sensitivity to perfumes and smoke, is a familiar hurdle. Join me as we explore the intersection of asthma with daily life, offering practical insights and empowering guidance for individuals and their caregivers.

What Climate is Best for a Person with Asthma?

Picture this: a gentle breeze rustling through leaves, carrying the scent of fresh air. For many with asthma, such serene scenes can be a breath of relief. In the quest for an ideal climate, consider these factors:

The Allure of Mildness: Generally, mild and temperate climates are more forgiving for individuals with asthma. Extreme temperatures, whether too hot or too cold, can sometimes trigger symptoms. A climate with moderate temperatures and lower humidity often provides a comfortable backdrop for easier breathing.

The Coastal Symphony: Coastal areas, with their crisp sea air, can be particularly inviting. The salt-laden breeze may have a beneficial impact on respiratory function. However, individual responses vary, so it's essential to pay attention to personal comfort.

Are Relaxing Exercises Good for My Asthma?

Enter the world of calming exercises, where the rhythm of breath and the stillness of the mind intertwine. For individuals with asthma, relaxing exercises can be a gentle ally in the journey to well-being.

The Magic of Mindfulness: Practices like yoga and tai chi invite you to synchronize breath with movement, fostering a sense of mindfulness. These exercises promote relaxation, potentially reducing stress – a common trigger for asthma symptoms.

The Art of Breath Control: Techniques like pursed-lip breathing and diaphragmatic breathing can enhance lung function and improve breath control. These exercises, when incorporated into daily routines, can contribute to a more harmonious relationship with your respiratory system.

Is There a Good Breathing Technique to Use When My Asthma Symptoms Get Worse?

In the face of worsening symptoms, having a toolbox of effective breathing techniques can make a significant difference. Consider these techniques to weather the storm:

Pursed-Lip Breathing: Picture yourself gently blowing through pursed lips, as if cooling a cup of hot tea. This technique slows down your breathing and helps keep airways open longer, making exhalation more effective.

Diaphragmatic Breathing: Place one hand on your chest and the other on your abdomen. As you breathe in, focus on allowing your abdomen to expand. This diaphragmatic breathing helps engage the diaphragm fully, enhancing the efficiency of your breath.

Deep Belly Breaths: In moments of distress, taking deep breaths can be a simple yet powerful remedy. Inhale deeply through your nose, allowing your belly to rise, and exhale slowly through your mouth. Repeat this process to create a calming rhythm.

How Does Asthma Affect My Choice of a Professional Career?

Life is a journey, and choosing a professional path involves considering various factors, including how asthma fits into the equation.

The Versatility of Careers: The good news is that asthma need not dictate your career choices. Many professions offer flexibility and accommodations to support individuals with asthma. Understanding your triggers and communicating your needs with employers can create a conducive work environment.

Remote Opportunities: In the digital age, remote work has become increasingly prevalent. This opens up a world of possibilities, allowing individuals with asthma to choose career paths that align with their health needs. The ability to work from the comfort of home can be a game-changer.

Building a Supportive Network: Surrounding yourself with a supportive network, including understanding colleagues and employers, is crucial. Open communication about your asthma and any accommodations you may require fosters a collaborative and inclusive workplace.

Sometimes People Have Trouble Understanding That I Can't Cope with Perfumes and Smoke. What Can I Do?

In a world scented with perfumes and veiled in smoke, navigating the challenges of sensitivities can be a delicate dance. Here's a guide to help clear the air:

Educate and Advocate: Often, people may not fully grasp the impact of perfumes and smoke on individuals with asthma. Take the opportunity to educate friends, family, and colleagues about your condition. Advocacy can foster understanding and empathy.

Set Boundaries: It's perfectly acceptable to communicate your boundaries when it comes to exposure to perfumes and smoke. Politely but firmly express your needs, whether it's requesting fragrance-free environments or kindly asking someone to smoke away from your vicinity.

Carry a Rescue Plan: Always have your rescue inhaler on hand. In situations where exposure is unavoidable, having a plan to manage potential symptoms is crucial. Consult with your healthcare team to ensure you're well-prepared.

What Can I Do to Improve My Home Environment in General?

Home is not just a place; it's a sanctuary for your well-being. Transforming your living space into an asthma-friendly haven involves a blend of practical adjustments and mindful choices.

The Air You Breathe: Invest in high-quality air purifiers to filter out common asthma triggers like dust mites and pet dander. Regularly clean and replace air filters in your heating and cooling systems to ensure the air circulating in your home is fresh and clean.

Dust Busters: Adopt dust-minimizing strategies, such as using allergen-proof mattress and pillow covers, regularly washing bedding in hot water, and keeping surfaces clutter-free to reduce dust accumulation.

Green Allies: Introduce indoor plants like aloe vera, spider plants, or peace lilies, which not only add a touch of nature but can also help improve air quality by absorbing certain pollutants.

Can I Have Pets Even Though I Have Asthma?

The pitter-patter of paws and the warm companionship of pets can bring immeasurable joy. The good news is, having asthma doesn't necessarily mean bidding farewell to furry friends.

The Pet Dilemma: While some individuals with asthma may be sensitive to pet allergens, others may find that their symptoms are well-managed with proper care. Regular grooming, keeping pets out of bedrooms, and investing in air purifiers can help minimize potential triggers.

Hypoallergenic Options: Consider breeds that are considered hypoallergenic, as they produce fewer allergens. Poodles, Bichon Frises, and certain types of terriers are among the breeds known for being more compatible with individuals with asthma.

When I Went to Spain on Holiday, I Felt Great – Should I Move There?

The allure of a different climate can be tantalizing, especially if a change in surroundings seems to bring relief. However, the decision to move should be approached with thoughtful consideration.

The Spanish Serenade: Spain's Mediterranean climate, with its warm, dry summers, is indeed appealing to many with asthma. The dry air and lower humidity can create a more comfortable environment for breathing. Before contemplating a move, it's advisable to spend an extended period in the desired location to gauge its long-term impact on your asthma.

Personal Climate Preferences: While some individuals with asthma may find relief in dry climates, others may fare better in more humid environments. It's a highly individualized experience, and understanding your personal preferences and triggers is key to making informed decisions.

My Asthma Means That I Have to Miss Out on Activities That Are Important to Me, Such as Dancing. This Makes Me Sad and Angry. What Can I Do?

The emotional toll of missing out on activities that bring joy can be profound. Acknowledging and addressing these feelings is an essential aspect of managing the emotional aspects of asthma.

Express and Release: Give yourself the space to express your emotions. Whether it's through journaling, talking to a friend, or engaging in creative outlets, acknowledging and releasing your feelings can be cathartic.

Adapt and Embrace: Explore modified versions of activities you love. While traditional dancing may pose challenges, consider alternative forms of movement like seated dance, gentle yoga, or tai chi. These adaptations allow you to stay connected to the activities that bring you joy while accommodating your respiratory needs.

Seek Support: Joining support groups or connecting with others who navigate similar challenges can provide a sense of community and understanding. Sharing experiences and coping strategies with others can be both comforting and empowering.

As we conclude this chapter, remember that your home is more than walls and furniture; it's a canvas for your well-being. From the air you breathe to the choices you make, every element plays a role in creating a supportive environment for asthma management.

Chapter 12
Author's Message

Dear Reader,

As I write this final chapter, I find myself reflecting on the journey we've taken together through the pages of this book. It has been a privilege to share this space with you, a space where we explored the intricacies of living with asthma and the myriad ways to not only cope but thrive.

Living with asthma is undoubtedly a challenge. It can feel like an unpredictable journey, a road with twists and turns that sometimes catch us off guard. I want you to know that it's okay to feel that way. This book is not just a collection of facts; it's a testament to the resilience that resides within you and the countless others who share this path.

Asthma doesn't distinguish between age, background, or circumstance. It touches lives indiscriminately, and in acknowledging this shared experience, we find strength. You are not alone in your journey. Millions around the world face similar challenges, and their stories intersect with yours, forming a tapestry of shared strength and perseverance.

Knowledge, as they say, is power. Throughout these pages, we've delved into the mechanics of asthma, its triggers, and various strategies for management. My hope is that this newfound knowledge empowers you, turning you into the captain of your own ship. This is not just about managing symptoms; it's about taking charge of your life.

Beyond inhalers and medications, we've explored the holistic aspects of well-being. Lifestyle, diet, exercise, and mental health all play crucial roles in the asthma journey. Small changes, made consistently, can yield significant results. It's a flexible journey, not a set of rigid rules.

To the caregivers reading this, your role is pivotal, and your support is immeasurable. Together, we've discussed how caregivers can be more than just providers of care; they can be partners in creating an environment where the challenges of asthma are met with understanding, compassion, and unwavering support.

As we conclude this book, I want to leave you with a message of hope. Asthma may be daunting, but it does not define your destiny. With each turn of the page, I've aimed to infuse hope – hope that each day brings a breath of fresh air, a step towards better control, and a realization of the incredible strength that resides within you.

This book is a tool, a resource, and a friend. It's not a substitute for professional medical advice, but rather a companion in your journey towards a fulfilling life despite asthma's presence.

Dear reader, I invite you to close this book with an open heart and a curious mind. Let's navigate the world of asthma together, armed with knowledge, surrounded by support, and buoyed by the hope that every breath brings us closer to a life lived to the fullest.

With warm regards,
KSK.